Fang Xiang Liao Fa

Essential Oil Analogues of TCM Herbal Formula

Esther E Aldrich
Randall R Bornemann

PUBLICATION NOTE:

Although we had interest from a number of publishers, we have decided to self-publish this book at this time. While we may go the more conventional route in the future, we felt it was important to keep costs low for our readers. We want to make this book accessible to you. We hope that, although the book might not be the fanciest volume on your shelf, the substantiveness of the content will help to make up for the plainness of its appearance.

REQUEST FOR FEEDBACK

We consider this to be a "beta" edition of the book. As self-publishing authors, we do not have access to professional copy editors. If you find errata, please notify us. Further, if you have ideas, suggestions or requests, also feel free to contact us. This book does not belong to us as authors. It belongs to the greater community of TCM practitioners and their patients. Is the binding holding up? Are we missing out on some of the subtle nuances of the TCM herbal formulas? Perhaps you'd like to tell us about some essential oils we haven't listed. Drop us a line! We'd love to hear from you.

tcmrandall@yahoo.com

Esther's Forward

Well here it is, **Fang Xiang Liao Fa**. We hope you like it and find it useful. What began as a personal quest for wellness has culminated in this project. We would never have laid this all out like this in systematic form if it wasn't for the interest from all our friends and colleagues. We would like to thank you all for your help and encouragement not only in our personal quests for wellness but in the research and development of this project. We couldn't have done this without each and every one of you.

First of all, we decided to keep the common names for each formula, rather than changing each suffix to the pinyin of "blend" ("Hun He Wu") or "essential oil blend" ("Xiang Jing You"). We are not fluent in Mandarin, and we just felt that keeping the commonly used names of the blends would be easier and keep things as clear as possible for people attempting to use the book.

You will note that there are certain oils we prefer to use more often than others. For yin, we will usually use Rose, Ylang Ylang and Jasmine. For spleen qi, we prefer Patchouli and Ginger. As a general yang tonic, our first choices will be Cinnamon and Ginger. These are just our preferences. We like these oils for their functions and indications, but they are also common oils and most of them have few if any cautions.

Preferred carrier oils include Sesame (nourish yin), Walnut (yang), Hazelnut (qi), Olive (blood), Safflower (move blood) and Jojoba (spleen qi/drain damp.) For exogenous conditions, we will usually use Sweet Almond, although Bitter Almond is useful for dispersing lung qi. Carrier oils can be high maintenance though. Keep in mind they are of secondary importance to the blend. Use what you have.

We have included thermal properties for most of the carriers, but the reader should bear in mind that it is the essential oils themselves that are going to account for most of the effects in that regard. Again, use what you have. It is more important to make sure the blend is properly diluted than it is to have the exact right carrier oil. If you have the recommended carrier, so much the better.

If you would like more in-depth information about the essential oils, we recommend **Jeffrey Yuen's** excellent Materia Medica. Our list was based on his, but expands upon it. He gives more information on the oils than we do. We just boil each one down to functions and indications. **Dennis Wilmont**'s website has some great information as well.

A great deal of thanks goes to our great friend and mentor **Soke W. Kent Bergstrom**. His background in pharmacology, chemistry and herbalism has been an often tapped well of useful information. His understanding of TCM, Eastern culture and the more esoteric and intuitive elements of our practice has been indispensable Likewise, his sense of humor more than once lightened up two overzealous students.

I would also like to thank my **Sifu Master Gin Foon Mark** who loved me like a father and was always encouraging to my endeavors in the Eastern arts. His understanding of the energetic anatomy, physics, biomechanics and herbs let me see the body more synergistically and holistically.

I can't go without mentioning **Dr. Brian Briggs** who was not only a selfless doctor, but a kindhearted mentor. He fed every question I had with a book and introduced me to TCM despite being an MD himself. He wrote my recommendation for grad school. Without him I'd never have travelled this path and probably would have died from undiagnosed thyroid disease. I am deeply indebted to you and you are sorely missed.

A special thank you to **Dr. Yubin Lu, Dr. Daiyi Tang**, and **Dr. Hong Chen** for spending so many extra hours with me teaching me how to compound herbal formulas and then correcting the formulas I would create.

Despite my background in English and love for it, I am overwhelmingly grateful to **Lousene Hoppe** who tirelessly edited this book so that I didn't compulsively edit it to death myself.

A lot of thanks also goes to my co-author **Randall Bornemann**, who wouldn't let me quit on this project. Through all the exhaustion, frustration and complications; this book made it to print and that is due mostly to him. I couldn't have and wouldn't have done it without you.

To my **mother** who has been my biggest fan, who tells me every time I talk to her how much she loves me and generally regards all my unconventional ideas with great interest: thank you. I couldn't ask for a better mom.

For my **dad**: I know it was hard for you to see me move off to another state and spend six years buried under a pile of books learning a medicine you had really never heard of. I know it was hard for you since to see how much debt my degree racked up. I know you worried if I'd ever make it. Thank you for letting me go out and try my hand at this and being so willing to help me out financially when student loans weren't enough and even still when their repayment threatens to break the bank.

Uncle Kyle, thank you for never once letting me try to be like anyone else. Thank you for constantly reassuring me that it was ok and good to just be me.

Reina, you would never let me be anything but the best. You've shown me I'm stronger than I think and helped me find the softness I almost lost in his hard world.

Robin, your devotion and dedication to me developing my practice is greatly appreciated. I am often reminded of the story of the turtle on the fencepost; none of us get where we are without help.

And finally, for all my grandparents:

Grandpa Ross, you always understood me when no one else did. You had a keen sense of my heart and always strove to nurture it, even when it spawned crazy art projects or neon red hair. I only wish you were still here to see how I've grown.

Grandma Thelma, you insist on paying me every time I treat you. You're so very intuitive and would always pay such close attention to the needs of others so much so that oftentimes you would already have what was needed without being asked. I've striven to learn this from you and incorporate it into my practice. In a world that is hardwired to appreciating linear and left brained activity you've helped me nurture the right brain that would have otherwise starved.

Grandma Stella, you are both honest and driven. You raised 5 boys and got a degree when even caucasian women were still not admitted to most universities much less Mexican women. You showed me I can achieve if I try. You showed me a woman can do everything, and you were always an open book. You are upfront and honest about what you think and feel. This taught me how to speak for myself and show myself to the world.

Grandpa Les, no one can survive as well as you can. You made it through the worst of WWII being in both Merrill's Marauders as well as in combat at Normandy. You taught me that I can survive anything. And even though you are tough, you still had enough softness to show me how to tend a garden with flowers and vegetables, how to make almost anything with a decent table saw, and how to use everything as an opportunity to teach (like the time I accidentally broke the curtain rod in your van, and instead of getting upset you just showed me how to fix it). I am resourceful to this day because of you.

To every friend, family member and patient who has supported, encouraged and nurtured me: thank you. Know that even if I didn't mention you by name, you are in my heart. I hope you like this book. It was made possible by all of you.

Esther Aldrich
January 2013

Randall's Forward

It looks like we're finally done! Thanks everyone for your curiosity, encouragement and suggestions. This whole thing started out as our own quest for wellness and has really blossomed into a whole new modality. I trust it will continue to grow now that we have finally provided a way to share it with everyone.

There are many people like us, who have sensitivity to many herbs due to their gluten content. There are many people, children for instance, who simply don't like needles. We offer a whole new treatment approach within the framework of TCM.

We're not Grand Masters of TCM. We're just students. Much of what we do is based upon experimentation and supposition. Yes, our work is based upon that of Masters like **Jeffrey Yuen** and **Soke W. Kent Bergstrom**. But we ourselves do not claim to be infallible.

This is especially true of the section on carrier oils. Many of these substances do have references in TCM literature, from the standpoint of herbology or dietary therapy. But there are also a few where we found ourselves trying to interpret Western functions and indications from the standpoint of TCM. So by all means, keep in touch! We want to hear from you! What are your experiences? Do you agree or disagree with us?

We look at this as a new modality, but it does not belong to us. It belongs to the greater community of TCM practitioners. We thank you for your interest, continuing questions, suggestions and ideas. It is from having to answer questions that we really began to develop a systematic methodology in our use of essential oils. We are grateful for all our friends and teachers in the TCM community, without whom we would never have rigorously formalized our approach.

I would especially like to thank my co-author, **Esther Aldrich. Esther** will stop at nothing in the pursuit of wellness, not only for herself but for her patients as well. Just being around her makes me stronger. Her commitment to healing others is exceeded only by her ingenuity and the depth of her research. I've learned tremendously from her, become a better healer, and I will always cherish the memories of working with her.

Randall Bornemann
January 2013

TABLE OF CONTENTS

Introduction to Essential Oils in TCM...1
    -Diluting Essential Oils...2
    -Testing the Oils..3
    -Top, Middle and Base Notes..4
    -Creating Blends..4
Application Techniques..7
Cautions and Contraindications...10
Suggested Points...12
Alphabetical Listing of Carrier Oils..15
MateriaMedica of Carrier Oils by Function and Indication..................................23
Alphabetical Listing of Essential Oils...37
MateriaMedica: Essential Oils by Function and Indications................................51
    -Astringe..53
    -Bi Syndrome...54
    -Calm the Shen..57
    -Clear Heat..60
    -Cool the Blood..65
    -Drain Damp..67
    -Food Stagnation...70
    -Invigorate Blood...72
    -Nourish Blood...76
    -Nourish Yin..78
    -Open Orifice...81
    -Parasites...82
    -Regulate Qi..85
    -Release the Exterior...89
    -Resolve Phlegm..93
    -Smooth Liver Qi...95
    -Spleen Qi...99
    -Stop Cough...104
    -Subdue Wind..106
    -Tonify Qi..107
    -Tonify Yang..112
    -Warm Interior to Expel Cold...115
    -Wei Qi..117

-**Ba Zhen Tang** (Eight-Treasure Decoction)
-**Ba Zheng San** (Eight-Herb Powder for Rectification)
-**Bai He Gu Jin Tang** (Lily Bulb Decoction to Preserve the Metal)
-**Bai Hu Tang** (White Tiger Decoction)
-**Bai Tou Weng Tang** (Pulsatilla Decoction)
-**Ban Xia Bai Zhu Tian Ma Tang** (Pinellia, Atractylodis Macrocephalae, and GastrodiaDecoction)
-**Ban Xia Hou Po Tang** (Pinellia and Magnolia Bark Decoction)
-**Ban Xia XieXin Tang** (Pinellia Decoction to Drain the Epigastrium)
-**Bao He Wan** (Preserve Harmony Pill)
-**Bu Yang Huan Wu Tang** (Tonify the Yang to Restore Five (Tenths) Decoction)
-**Bu Zhong Yi Qi Tang** (Tonify the Middle and Augment the Qi Decoction)
-**Cang Er Zi San** (Xanthium Powder)
-**Chai Ge Jie Ji Tang** (Bupleurum and Kudzu Decoction)
-**Chai Hu Shu Gan San** (Bupleurum Powder to Spread the Liver)
-**Chuan Xiong Cha Tiao San** (LigusticumChuanxiong Powder)
-**Da Bu Yin Wan** (Great Tonify the Yin Pill)
-**Da Chai Hu Tang** (Major Bupleurum Decoction)
-**Da Cheng Qi Tang** (Major Order the Qi Decoction)
-**Da Jian Zhong Tang** (Major Construct the Middle Decoction)
-**Dang Gui Bu Xue Tang** (Tangkuei Decoction to Tonify the Blood)
-**Dang Gui Liu Huang Tang** (Tangkuei and Six-Yellow Decoction)
-**Dao Chi San** (Guide Out the Red Powder)
-**Ding Chuan Tang** (Arrest Wheezing Decoction)
-**Du HuoJi Sheng Tang** (Angelica Pubescens and Sangjisheng Decoction)
-**Du Qi Wan** (Capital Qi Pill)
-**Er Chen Tang** (Two-Cured Decoction)
-**Er Miao San** (Two Marvel Powder)
-**Er Xian Tang** (Two-Immortal Decoction)
-**ErZhi Wan** (Two-Ultimate Pill)
-**Fu Yuan HuoXue Tang** (Revive Health by Invigorating the Blood Decoction)
-**Gan Mai Da Zao Tang** (Licorice, Wheat, and Jujube Decoction)
-**Gan Mao Ling** (Miraculous Medicine for Cold and Flu)
-**Ge Gen Huang Lian Huang Qin Tang** (Kudzu, Coptis, and ScutellariaDecoction)
-**Ge Gen Tang** (Kudzu Decoction)

-**Ge Xia Zhu Yu Tang** (Drive Out Blood Stasis Below the Diaphragm Decoction)
-**Gui Pi Tang** (Restore the Spleen Decoction)
-**Gui Zhi Shao Yao Zhi Mu Tang** (Cinnamon Twig, Peony, and Anemarrhena Decoction)
-**Gui Zhi Tang** (Cinnamon Twig Decoction)
-**Gui Zhi Fu Ling Wan** (Cinnamon Twig and Poria Pill)
-**Huang Lian E Jiao Tang** (Coptis and Ass-Hide Gelatin Decoction)
-**Huang Lian Jie Du Tang** (Coptis Decoction to Relieve Toxicity)
-**Huo Xiang Zheng Qi San** (Agastache Powder to Rectify the Qi)
-**Ji Chuan Jian** (Benefit the River (Flow) Decoction)
-**Jiao Ai Tang** (Ass-Hide Gelatin and Mugwort Decoction)
-**Jin Gui Shen Qi Wan** (Kidney Qi Pill from the Golden Cabinet)
-**Jin Suo Gu Jing Wan** (Metal Lock Pill to Stabilize the Essence)
-**Ju Pi Zhu Ru Tang** (Tangerine Peel and Bamboo Shaving Decoction)
-**Juan Bi Tang** (Remove Painful Obstruction Decoction)
-**Li Zhong Wan** (Regulate the Middle Pill)
-**Ling Gui Zhu Gan Tang** (Poria, Cinnamon Twig, Atractylodis Macrocephalae and Licorice Decoction)
-**Ling Jiao Gou Teng Tang** (Antelope Horn and Uncaria Decoction)
-**Liu Wei Di Huang Wan** (Six-Ingredient Pill with Rehmannia)
-**Long Dan XieGan Tang** (GentianaLongdancao Decoction to Drain the Liver)
-**Ma Huang Tang** (Ephedra Decoction)
-**Ma Xing Yi Gan Tang** (Ephedra Apricot Kernel Coicis and Licorice Decoction)
-**Ma Xing Shi Gan Tang** (Ephedra, Apricot Kernel, Gypsum and Licorice Decoction)
-**Ma Zi Ren Wan** (Hemp Seed Pill)
-**Mai Men Dong Tang** (Ophiopogonis Decoction)
-**Mu Li San** (Oyster Shell Powder)
-**Nuan Gan Jian** (Warm the Liver Decoction)
-**Ping Wei San** (Calm the Stomach Powder)
-**Pu Ji Xiao Du Yin** (Universal Benefit Decoction to Eliminate Toxin)
-**Qi Ju Di Huang Wan** (LyciumRehmanniaTeapills)
-**Qiang Huo Sheng Shi Tang** (Notopterygium Decoction to Overcome Dampness)
-**Qing Gu San** (Cool the Bones Powder)
-**Qing Hao Bie Jia Tang** (Artemisia Annua and Soft-Shelled Turtle Shell Decoction)

-**Qing Qi Hua Tan Wan** (Clear the Qi and Transform Phlegm Pill)
-**Qing Wei San** (Clear the Stomach Powder)
-**Qing Ying Tang** (Clear the Nutritive Level Decoction)
-**Qing Zao Jiu Fei Tang** (Eliminate Dryness and Rescue the Lungs Decoction)
-**Ren Shen Bai Du San** (Ginseng Powder to Overcome Pathogenic Influences)
-**San Zi Yang Qin Tang** (Three-Seed Decoction to Nourish One"s Parents)
-**Sang Ju Yin** (Mulberry Leaf and Chrysanthemum Decoction)
-**Sang Piao Xiao San** (Mantis Egg-Case Powder)
-**Sang Xing Tang** (Mulberry Leaf and Apricot Kernel Decoction)
-**Shao Fu Zhu Yu Tang** (Drive-Out Blood Stasis in the Lower Abdomen)
-**Shao Yao Tang** (Peony Decoction)
-**Shen Ling Bai Zhu San** (Ginseng, Poria and Atractylodes Macrocephala Powder)
-**Shen Tong Zhu Yu Tang** (Drive Out Blood Stasis from a Painful Body Decoction)
-**Sheng Hua Tang** (Generation and Transformation Decoction)
-**Sheng Mai San** (Generate the Pulse Powder)
-**Shi Quan Da Bu Tang** (All Inclusive Great Tonifying Decoction)
-**Shi Xiao San** (Sudden Smile Powder)
-**Si Jun Zi Tang** (Four-Gentleman Decoction)
-**Si Ni San** (Frigid Extremities Powder)
-**Si Shen Wan** (Four-Miracle Pill)
-**Si Wu Tang** (Four-Substance Decoction)
-**Su Zi Jiang Qi Tang** (Perilla Fruit Decoction for Directing Qi Downward)
-**Suan Zao Ren Tang** (Sour Jujube Decoction)
-**Tian Ma Gou Teng Yin** (Gastrodia and Uncaria Decoction)
-**Tian Tai Wu Yao San** (Top-quality Lindera Powder)
-**Tian Wang Bu Xin Dan** (Emperor of Heaven's Special Pill to Tonify the Heart)
-**Tiao Wei Cheng Qi Tang** (Regulate the Stomach and Order the Qi Decoction)
-**Tong Xie Yao Fang** (Important Formula for Painful Diarrhea)
-**Wan Dai Tang** (End Discharge Decoction)
-**Wen Dan Tang** (Warm the Gallbladder Decoction)
-**Wen Jing Tang** (Warm the Menses Decoction)
-**Wu Ling San** (Five-Ingredient Powder with Poria)
-**Wu Pi San** (Five-Peel Powder)

-Wu Wei Xiao Du Yin (Five-Ingredient Decoction to Eliminate Toxin)
-Wu Zhu Yu Tang (Evodia Decoction)
-Xiao Chai Hu Tang (Minor Bupleurum Decoction)
-Xiao Cheng Qi Tang (Minor Order the Qi Decoction)
-Xiao Feng San (Eliminate Wind Powder from True Lineage)
-Xiao Jian Zhong Tang (Minor Construct the Middle Decoction)
-Xiao Qing Long Tang (Minor Blue-Green Dragon Decoction)
-Xiao Yao San (Rambling Powder)
-Xie Bai San (Drain the White Powder)
-Xie Xin Tang (Drain the Epigastrium Decoction)
-Xi Jiao Di Huang Tang (Rhinoceros Horn and Rehmannia Decoction)
-Xing Su San (Apricot Kernel and Perilla Leaf Powder)
-Xue Fu Zhu Yu Tang (Drive Out Stasis in the Mansion of Blood Decoction)
-Yi Guan Jian (Linking Decoction)
-Yin Chen Hao Tang (Artemisia Yinchenhao Decoction)
-Yin Qiao San (Honeysuckle and Forsythia Powder)
-You Gui Wan (Restore the Right (Kidney) Pill)
-You Gui Yin (Restore the Right Kidney Decoction)
-Yu Nu Jian (Jade Woman Decoction)
-Yu Ping Feng San (Jade Windscreen Powder)
-Yue Ju Wan (Escape Restraint Pill)
-Zhen Gan Xi Feng Tang (Sedate the Liver and Extinguish Wind Decoction)
-Zhen Wu Tang (True Warrior Decoction)
-Zhi Bai Di Huang Tang (AnemarrhenaPhellodendron and Rehmannia Decoction)
-Zhi Gan Cao Tang (Honey-Fried Licorice Decoction)
-Zhi Sou San (Stop Coughing Powder)
-Zhu Ling Tang (Polyporus Decoction)
-Zhu Ye Shi Gao Tang (Lophatherus and Gypsum Decoction)
-Zou Gui Wan (Restore the Left Kidney Pill)
-Zuo Jin Wan (Left Metal Pill)

Bibliography...253
Appendix: Chemistry of Essential Oils...254

INTRODUCTION TO THE USE OF ESSENTIAL OILS IN TRADITIONAL CHINESE MEDICINE

Welcome to **Fang Xiang Liao Fa: Essential Oil Analogues of TCM Herbal Formulas.** We would like to start out by saying that there is no "right" or "wrong" way to use these oils. Aside from general safety precautions, of course. This is, to some degree, unexplored territory. Unlike in herbology, where there is general consensus on what herbs constitute the traditional formulas, the use of essential oils is fairly wide open.

In fact, there really is no hard and fast list of functions and indications for these oils, from a TCM standpoint. This was the biggest obstacle in our research. Thankfully there are a few excellent sources out there, like **Jeffrey Yuen**'s Materia Medica. Our list is based upon his, but expands on it. We would like to state from the outset, that if you disagree with us on some of these functions, indications, or anything else for that matter, please feel free to do so. We are all in the process of learning.

With that said, we wanted to share with everyone the way we do things. There has been a great deal of curiosity as to what we do and how we do it. That's what this is, a book on how we do things. Take it as your starting point, especially when it comes to the blends themselves. But don't be limited by it.

Our goal with these blends was to reproduce the sets of functions and indications of the traditional herbal formulas. We mainly do this by using the most common and safest oils. But given our Materia Medica, there are many other blends and combinations that could be used. Some will work better for some people, while others will work better for others. Some people may have allergies to or preferences for certain fragrances.

The goal is not to imitate what we do by rote, but to make the art and science your own.

Diluting Essential Oils

We always dilute the oils. Sometimes people will tell you to apply them "neat." That means to apply them directly to the skin without dilution. We don't do that. We mix the oils with a carrier oil. This dilutes the oils significantly, however the oils are quite powerful. You will still have an effective blend even with just a few drops of the oil.

The general dosage in our blends is 30 drops of essential oil per ounce of carrier oil. However, we generally don't make a whole ounce at a time. We normally use roller bottles, which are small cylindrical bottles with a plastic roller on the end, and contain about 1/3 of an ounce. Therefore our blends will usually contain approximately 10 drops of essential oil and 1/3 oz of carrier.

We find that this is a good amount to give the the patient, as we don't want to give them an amount that will last longer than they need the formula. This might result in self-medicating, even after the point at which they should switch to a different blend. We also feel that the roller bottles are a convenient way to apply the oils, although the plastic roller does not mix well with some oils. A glass rod would be ideal in that case.

Adult Dose:
30 drops to 1 oz.
10 drops to 1/3 oz.

For children, we will reduce the dosage, depending upon how much they weigh. Generally for children 6 and under, use maybe 3 drops, or 1/3 of the regular dosage, whereas for older children through puberty, use half an adult dosage. For babies and very small children, it may not even be necessary to apply the oils directly to the skin. You can apply them to your fingers and hold them over the points into which you would like to direct qi. Visualize qi flowing through your fingers and onto the points. However the general modality is in applying them in a diluted form to points and/or using them in pediatric Tui Na.

Very small children:
10 drops to 1 oz.
3 drops to 1/3 oz

Older Children:
15 drops to 1 oz.
5 drops to 1/3 oz.

We will also halve the dosage when applying oils to the head, especially sensitive points like Yintang.

Testing the Oils

We always test the oils before we use them. Some patients will be sensitive to certain oils. Sometimes this can come as a surprise. People with no history of allergies can have reactions to essential oils.

Before applying the oils therapeutically, try them in small amounts on the soles of the feet. Use a carrier oil to wipe the oil off the feet if necessary. Oils do not mix with water. If for some reason, you can't test the oils on the soles of the feet, try the inside of the upper arm.

Keep this in mind if you get oils in your eye. From time to time you will get oils on your hands. If you scratch your face or in particular your eyes, you will spread these oils into sensitive areas. Using water can make this worse, so you really want to use a carrier oil.

It should be noted that you don't necessarily want to come into contact with the oils. This could have a similar effect as taking a small dosage of all the herbs you prescribe throughout the day. It can add up. You also may subsequently have a patient who reacts to those fragrances or develop a sensitization yourself. Only apply oils to yourself if you are using them for yourself. Avoid taking other peoples' prescriptions.

Top, Middle and Base Notes

Essential oils are divided into three categories, based upon how rapidly they evaporate. These are top notes, middle notes and base notes.

Top notes last 2-4 hours.
Middle notes last approximately 6 hours.
Base notes last 1-2 days.

We believe these "notes" also correspond roughly to the three jiao of the human body. **Jeffrey Yuen** corresponds them to different levels in the body, as far as Wei Qi, Yin Qi and Yuan Qi. You can look at it from that perspective too. However essential oils are the "Jing Essence" of the plant. We believe they provide "Yuan Qi" to whatever points and meridians to which they are applied.

Creating Blends

Many times the blends we create will not exactly match the functions and indications of any specific herbal formula. We do provide essential oil versions of the formulas here, but our purpose is not to limit the practitioner, but to offer examples or suggestions as to how one might go about creating blends. Don't be afraid to experiment or deviate from the prescriptions we lay out.

Jeffrey Yuen formulates blends differently than we do. His idea is to use base notes for the "monarch" oil, and to use middle and top notes for the secondary functions and indications. Professor Yuen seems to suggest that his blends will generally have one oil of each note, top, bottom and base. We have a different method.

We will generally use one, two or sometimes three (occasionally more) oils in our blends, but we generally use all oils of the same note. Generally for chronic, constitutional issues, we will use base notes. For digestive issues and issues pertaining to the middle jiao, we will tend to use middle notes. And for exogenous pathogens, we will sometimes use top notes.

This way, we can apply the blends more frequently if necessary. If we are using a base note, we don't necessarily want to reapply the oil more than once a day. However, if we are using middle notes, we can apply the blend every 6 hours. This way, all the oils in the formula are working, and we don't have to worry about one or two of them evaporating before the other. One exception to this rule is in clearing empty heat. In that case, we might use base notes to nourish yin, but then middle notes to clear heat.

Another exception might be if we do not have another oil of that note available. If we are looking for a base note, but we do not have one, we will go with a middle note if necessary. In that case we could try to make the whole blend of middle notes and just apply it more frequently. Base note formulas are good, because the patient may not want to have to apply the oils more than once a day.

Generally speaking, we will try to use as few oils as possible. If one oil hits all of our functions and indications, we will use just that oil (with a carrier, of course.) Most of our blends will consist of two essential oils and one carrier. A few consist of three or more essential oils. We will also tend to use oils that are the most common, and also that are the safest. For example, if we need an oil to regulate qi, we would tend to select the oil that has fewer cautions and contraindications.

One last issue is harmonizing the blends. In herbology, we will generally use Gan Cao, or Licorice Root to harmonize the herbs in the formula. In using essential oils, it is not necessary to use a harmonizer like that. The carrier oil will harmonize the formula.

However, if you want to try an oil that will harmonize a blend, **Jeffrey Yuen** recommends Ginger and Ho leaf. Ginger is warming, whereas Ho Leaf is cooling. They are both middle notes, although Ginger is also a base note. (It can be used as either a middle or a base note.) Beyond that, you could try Galangal, which is a form of Ginger, or in general oils listed as tonifying spleen qi. These tend to be warming, so if you want something cooling, try one of the oils listed as smoothing liver qi.

We will generally create two versions of each blend. The functions and indications will be the same, but the oils will be different. This is to prevent sensitization. Sensitization occurs when a person develops an allergic reaction to an oil. This may result from overuse. This is why we dilute our oils. However, we also ask patients to switch blends every so often. If a patient tends to have allergies, we will ask them to use one version of the blend for 3 days, then switch to the other version, and back and forth, occasionally taking days off without applying the blends. If a patient has no history of allergies, maybe they can go 5 days before switching back and forth. But it's important not to use the same oils all the time.

Point Prescriptions

Anyone with training in TCM will be able to select points on which to apply the blends. However we do give a basic outline of suggested points. When we send patients home with a blend, we generally don't give them points on the back, as those points can be difficult to reach and locate. We'll mainly go with yuan source points and areas that are easy to find. Du 4 is an exception to this rule, as it is a cardinal point for tonifying yang. The oils do not have to be applied exactly on the point, they can be spread over the general area of the point. As long as that general area includes the point itself, this is usually fine.

Application Techniques

We usually use roller bottles, although a glass rod is ideal. The glass will not react with any of the oils. Oils high in phenols will tend to react with the plastic. You simply immerse one end of the glass rod into the oils, then apply them to the points. You can also use plastic guide tubes, although again, some of the oils will react with the plastic. Diluting the oils is one way to mitigate this phenomenon, but as always it is something to consider when selecting oils for a blend.

The techniques used in applying oils to points are based on the classical needling techniques.

Wei Qi

To apply oils for acute conditions, apply them in a circular motion. To tonify, you would apply them in a circular motion upwards and toward the center line of the body. To reduce, you would go upward and away from the center line of the body. On the center line of the body, you would apply them in a circular motion: clockwise to tonify, counter-clockwise to reduce. The circular motion will connect with the wei qi.

Diffuser: You can also put the oils in a diffuser and breathe them in the air. Do this for 20 minutes, no less than 2-3 hours apart. Diffusers will allow anyone in the room to benefit from the blend. This technique will rid the air of viruses, bacteria and "pathological qi."

You can also add the oils to boiling water and let it rise in the steam, or put 2-3 drops on the palms of your hands and inhale them.

Internal Conditions

For internal conditions, apply the oils by lifting and thrusting. You can also rub them in the direction of the channel, against the direction of the channel or you can hold the roller bottle or glass rod on the point and vibrate it. To rub them in the direction of the channel will tonify, to go against the channel will tend to reduce. Vibrating will connect with the yuan or constitutional level.

Lifting and Thrusting: Lifting and thrusting in application of essential oils is based on that of the needling technique. Emphasis on lifting will tend to reduce. Emphasis on thrusting will tend to tonify.

Direction of the Channel: This is similar to lifting or thrusting, only it is more applying them in a straight line in the direction of the channel, or against the direction of the channel. Applying the oils in the direction of the channel will tend to tonify, while pressing against the direction will tend to reduce.

Vibrating: This means holding the applicator onto a point and vibrating it on that point. This is more similar to a Tui Na or Medical QiGong technique. It is used to tonify on the yuan level.

You can also apply **DMSO (DiMethyl SulfOxide)** over the oils, to cause them to go extra deep into the point. This should be done with caution however, as **DMSO** is a strong carrier, and will carry anything that comes into contact with it deep into the body. **DMSO** also has a strong drying property. If you want to mitigate this drying property, use it mixed with aloe.

Other techniques include applying the oils to the points before needling to enhance the treatment effect or dipping the needles in the oils before needling. As always, the oils themselves would be selected to correspond to the functions and indications of the points, as well as the treatment goals.

Auricular application: You can apply oils to the microsystems of the ear or other parts of the body, such as the scalp, hands and feet. For this we will usually use rotating towards the centerline of the body to tonify, away to reduce, vibrating or possibly visualization of qi carrying the oil into the point. NOTE: As always, when applying a blend to the head, we will halve the dosage.

Other Techniques

Compress: Apply a few drops topically, then cover with a hot, moist towel. Cover this with a dry towel to lock in the heat. Do this until the hot towel cools down, or until the patient decides to quit. It shouldn't go more than an hour or so. For a compress, it is not necessary to dilute the oils in a carrier, as you are only using 2-3 drops.

For children, mix oils into some water, then as they float to the surface, soak them up in a towel. Use this towel as the compress. Wring it out and apply, covered with a dry towel. Do not scald the child or use too many drops of essential oils. We would use about 10 drops in a basin of water.

Bathing: You can mix about 3-4 drops of oil with a cup of epsom salts. Or you can use approximately 10 drops of oils in a bath gel.

To soak feet, use about 5-8 drops in a basin of warm water.

Suppositories: We do not use suppositories or vaginal injections of essential oils. You can make suppositories with Coconut butter as a medium.

Disinfectant

Occasionally we will use tea tree oil undiluted to swab points for acupuncture. This is due to the fact that isopropyl alcohol is carcinogenic. If you have a cancer patient, they may request an alternative to conventional alcohol swabs.

Cautions and Contraindications

-Make sure you are cognizant of the cautions and contraindications of the various oils.

-Many oils, especially citrus oils, can be photosensitive. Use them carefully if the skin is going to be exposed to the sun. This is especially true of tanning beds.

-Oils strong in menthol should not be used on children aged 3 and under. This includes peppermint, camphor, wintergreen, etc.

-Do not apply oils to the inner ear. If you are using the auricular microsystem, use only a very small amount so that there will not be a large enough drop to flow to the inner portion of the ear.

-We will halve the dosage of the blend if we use it on the auricular microsystem or anywhere on the head.

-Keep oils away from the eyes. If you have oils on your fingers, be mindful not to rub your eyes.

-Test the oils on the soles of the feet or on the inside of the upper arm region to make sure there will be no reaction. This is especially important in people who have allergies.

-If irritation occurs, dilute the oil on the skin with a carrier oil. We use corn oil. Water will not mix with the oil, and may exacerbate the situation.

-Keep oils out of reach of children. We do not take them internally at all. If an oil is ingested, dilute with milk and call poison control.

-Keep oils away from flames, sparks and sources of electricity. Some may be flammable.

-Do not add oils directly to bath water. First dilute with a carrier oil or a bath gel.

-Do not apply undiluted essential oils to mucous membranes.

-If a person has allergies, use caution in exposing them to the air in which a diffuser is being used. We will usually use the foot microsystem if a person has allergies. Do not apply them on the face or head of a person with allergies. If the allergies are severe or unpredictable, just don't use essential oils.

-Pregnant women, people diagnosed with epilepsy or seizure disorders and people with hypertension should consult a physician before using essential oils. This is also true in women who are nursing.

-Be mindful that some essential oils, like Clary Sage, have an estrogenic property. This may not be suitable, for instance, in the case of a patient with breast cancer.

-Use common sense.

-Adhere to basic TCM theory. If someone has a yang excess, do not exacerbate that with excessive yang oils.

-If you are treating multiple patients, limit exposure to essential oils, as some patients may be sensitive to them.

-If you are starting out using essential oils, make sure you drink plenty of water. You may experience a Herxheimer effect. This occurs when toxins are being released or expelled from the body. You may feel sick as a result of this process. Drinking water will help flush these toxins out and minimize the discomfort.

-Dilute the blend if you are using it on children.

Further Reading

Aromatherapy for Babies and Children by Shirley Price

Essential Oil Safety: A Guide for Health Care Professionals by Robert Tisserand

Suggested Points

Astringe
Sp 1, 3, Du 20

Bi syndrome
LI 4, Liv 3, Sp 10, Ashi

Calm the shen
Pc 6, Du 20, Yintang

Clear heat
LI 4, SJ 5, LI 11, Du 14

Cool the blood
Lu 9, Sp 10, LI 4, SJ 5, LI 11, Du 14

Drain damp
Sp 9, 3, 6, UB 20

Food stagnation
Ren 12, Pc 6, LI 4, Liv 3, St 25, 36, Sp 3

Invigorate blood
Sp 10, UB 17, Jiaji

Nourish blood
UB 17, Jiaji, Sp 3, 6, St 36, Kid 3

Nourish yin
Kid 3, UB 23, Ren 4, 6, Liv 3

Open orifice
Du 20, Pc 6, Ren 17

Parasites
St 25, Ren 4, LI 4

Regulate qi
LI 4, Liv 3

Release the exterior
LI 4, SJ 5, LI 11, Du 14

12Resolve phlegm
St 40, Sp 3, 6, 9

Smooth liver qi
Liv 2(excess), Liv 3(deficiency), LI 4, Sp 6

Spleen qi
Sp 3, 4, 6

Stop cough
Ren 17, Lung 7

Subdue wind
Liv 3, Du 14, GB 20

Tonify qi
Ren 17, Pc 6, St 36

Tonify yang
Du 4, St 36

Warm exterior to expel cold
Du 4, St 36, Ren 6

Wei qi
Lu 9, Ren 17, Sp 3

Carrier Oils
Alphabetical List

NOTE:

Many of the carrier oils listed have questions marks by them. This indicates situations in which the authors disagree as to the functions, indications or thermal properties of the oil. In some cases, the information is unknown. The questions marks refer to functions, indications or thermal properties that are in dispute.

CARRIER OILS

Acai (Nourish yin, Tonify qi)

Almond (sweet) N (Nourish yin/lung, Release the exterior, Resolve phlegm, Stop cough, Tonify qi/lung, Other: Regulates colon)

Almond (bitter) (Diffuses, Disperses lung qi)

Aloe Cold (Clear heat/liver fire, Nourish yin, Parasites, Other: Purges downward, Constipation)

Andiroba C (Nourish yin, Move qi and blood, Parasites, Spleen qi, Stop cough)

Apricot Kernel W (Stops cough, Other: Moistens Large Intestine, Purges downward)

Argan (Invigorate blood, Nourish yin? Wei qi)

Arnica C? (Move qi and blood)

Avocado C (Nourish blood, Nourish yin, Smoothes liver qi)

Babassu Palm C? (Astringe? Move qi and blood?)

Baobab (Nourish yin)

Black Cumin Seed (Tonify qi, Nourish yin, Spleen qi)

Black Raspberry Seed N (Astringe, Nourish blood, Nourish yin/kidney/liver)

Blackberry Seed N (Astringe, Nourish blood, Nourish yin/kidney, Spleen qi)

Black Currant Seed W? (Drain damp, Spleen Qi, Stop cough)

Borage C (Nourish blood, Nourish liver yin, Smooth liver qi)

Calendula C (Astringe, Food stagnation, Invigorate blood, Release exterior, Other: Promote menstruation)

Camelina (Green tea oil) C (Tonify qi/lung, Spleen qi, Other: Detoxify)

Camelia Seed C (Drain damp, Spleen qi)

Carrot N (Drain damp, Parasites, Resolve phlegm, Spleen qi)

Castor (Nourish yin, Parasites, Other: Purge Colon in constipation)

Centella Cold (Astringe, Clear heat, Drain damp, Cools the blood)

Chamomille C (Calm the shen, Clear heat, Dry damp, Subdue wind)

Cherry Kernel W (Astringe, Spleen qi, Tonify qi)

Cocoa Butter (Calms the shen, Drains damp)

Coconut W (Nourish yin/heart, Subdue wind)

Coffee, Green W (Drain damp, Nourish blood, Tonify yang/heart)

Coffee, Roasted W (Drain damp, Tonify yang/heart)

Cohune Nut (Nourish yin? Nourish blood?)

Copaiba (Drain damp)

Corn N (Drain damp, Nourish yin/heart/kidney, Spleen qi)

Cottonseed (Invigorate blood/lower, Yang tonic, Other: Induces abortion)

Cranberry Seed C (Clear heat, Drain damp)

Cucumber Seed C (Clear heat/Summerheat, Nourish yin, Parasites, Spleen qi)

Cumin Seed W (Regulate qi, Spleen qi)

Egg N (Nourish blood, Nourish yin, Spleen qi, Tonify qi)

Emu C (Move qi and blood, Nourish yin, Nourish blood)

Evening Primrose (Nourish blood, Nourish liver yin, Spleen qi)

Grapeseed C (Drain damp, Nourish yin, Tonify qi)

Hazelnut (Spleen qi, Tonify qi/Yuan qi)

Hemp Seed N (Nourish yin)

Jojoba (Drain damp, Resolve phlegm)

Karanja W (Bi syndrome, Invigorate blood, Nourish blood, Parasites)

Kukui Nut C (Nourish yin)

Lime Blossom C (Astringe, Calm the shen, Clear heat/summer heat, Cools the blood, Drain damp, Invigorates blood, Parasites, Resolve phlegm, Smoothes liver qi, Spleen qi)

Linseed (flax seed) N (Move qi and blood, Resolve phlegm, Spleen qi)

Macadamia (Nourish yin)

Manketti (Nourish yin, Tonify qi)

Mango Seed W (Nourish yin, Spleen qi)

Marula C (Drain damp, Nourish yin, Spleen qi)

Meadowfoam (Move blood)

Monoi N? (Drain damp, Nourish yin/heart, Subdue wind)

Moringa (Nourish blood, Nourish yin)

Mustard Seed W (Drain damp, Regulate qi, Resolve phlegm/lung, Spleen qi)

Neem C (Clear heat, Drain damp, Parasites, Other: Contraceptive)

Oat W (Nourish yin, Regulate qi, Spleen qi, Tonify qi)

Olive (Drain damp, Nourish blood)

Palm Kernal W (Nourish yin/heart, Subdue wind)

Papaya N (Drain damp, Spleen qi, Smooth liver qi)

Passion Flower (Calm the shen, Move qi and blood)

Peach Kernel C (Moves qi and blood, Other: Drain abcess, Moisten intestine to move bowel)

Peanut W (Astringe, Nourish yin/lung, Spleen qi, Stop cough)

Pecan (Wei qi)

Pequi

Perilla Seed W (Food stasis, Stop cough, Other: Moistens intestine to move bowel)

Pistachio N (Nourish yin, Tonify qi)

Plum Kernel C (Nourish yin/liver)

Pomace Olive (Drain damp, Nourish blood)

Pomegranite Seed C (Parasites)

Poppy Seed N (Move qi and blood/chest, Other: Contain lung qi, Bind large intestine)

Pracaxi

Pumpkin Seed N (Drain damp, Parasites, Spleen qi)

Rapeseed W (Regulate qi, Resolve phlegm)

Red Raspberry Seed N (Astringe, Nourish blood, Nourish yin/kidney/liver)

Rice Bran W (Spleen qi, Tonify qi)

Rose Hip W (Astringe, Drain damp, Tonify qi/kidney)

Safflower W (Invigorate blood, Other: Promote menstruation)

Sea Buckthorn (Move qi and blood, Nourish yin)

Sesame (Nourish blood, Nourish yin/Jing essence, Parasites)

Shea Butter (Move qi and blood?, Resolve phlegm)

Sisymbrium (Tonify qi)

Soy C (Clear heat, Drain damp, Invigorate blood, Nourish yin, Spleen qi)

St. John's Wort C (Astringe, Bi Syndrome, Clear heat, Smooth liver qi, Stop cough)

Sunflower W (Spleen qi, Tonify qi)

Tamanu C (Move qi and blood)

Walnut W (Tonify yang/kidney, Other: Helps kidneys grasp qi)

Watermelon Seed Cold (Clear heat, Drain damp)

Wheatgerm C (Calm the shen, Invigorate blood, Nourish yin)

Witch Hazel (Astringe, Calm the shen, Invigorate blood, Spleen qi, Tonify qi)

Yangu

Carrier Oils
Materia Medica

NOTE:

Many of the carrier oils listed have questions marks by them. This indicates situations in which the authors disagree as to the functions, indications or thermal properties of the oil. In some cases, the information is unknown. The questions marks refer to functions, indications or thermal properties that are in dispute.

Astringe

Babassu Palm C? (Astringe? Move qi and blood?)

Black Raspberry Seed N (Astringe, Nourish blood, Nourish yin/kidney/liver)

Blackberry Seed N (Astringe, Nourish blood, Nourish yin/kidney, Spleen qi)

Calendula C (Astringe, Food stagnation, Invigorate blood, Release exterior, Other: Promote mestruation)

Centella Cold (Astringe, Clear heat, Drain damp, Cools the blood)

Cherry Kernel W (Astringe, Spleen qi, Tonify qi)

Lime Blossom C (Astringe, Calm the shen, Clear heat/summer heat, Cools the blood, Drain damp, Invigorates blood, Parasites, Resolve phlegm, Smoothes liver qi, Spleen qi)

Peanut W (Astringe, Nourish yin/lung, Spleen qi, Stop cough)

Red Raspberry Seed N (Astringe, Nourish blood, Nourish yin/kidney/liver)

Rose Hip W (Astringe, Drain damp, Tonify qi/kidney)

St. John's Wort C (Astringe, Bi Syndrome, Clear heat, Smooth liver qi, Stop cough)

Witch Hazel (Astringe, Calm the shen, Invigorate blood, Spleen qi, Tonify qi)

Bi Syndrome

Karanja W (Bi syndrome, Invigorate blood, Nourish blood, Parasites)

St. John's Wort C (Astringe, Bi Syndrome, Clear heat, Smooth liver qi, Stop cough)

Calm the Shen

Chamomille C (Calm the shen, Clear heat, Dry damp, Subdue wind)

Cocoa Butter (Calms the shen, Drains damp)

Lime Blossom C (Astringe, Calm the shen, Clear heat/summer heat, Cools the blood, Drain damp, Invigorates blood, Parasites, Resolve phlegm, Smoothes liver qi, Spleen qi)

Passion Flower (Calm the shen, Move qi and blood)

Wheatgerm C (Calm the shen, Invigorate blood, Nourish yin)

Witch Hazel (Astringe, Calm the shen, Invigorate blood, Spleen qi, Tonify qi)

Clear Heat

Aloe Cold (Clear heat/liver fire, Nourish yin, Parasites, Other: Purges downward, Constipation)

Centella Cold (Astringe, Clear heat, Drain damp, Cools the blood)

Chamomille C (Calm the shen, Clear heat, Dry damp, Subdue wind)

Cranberry Seed C (Clear heat, Drain damp)

Cucumber Seed C (Clear heat/summerheat, Nourish yin, Parasites, Spleen qi)

Lime Blossom C (Astringe, Calm the shen, Clear heat/summer heat, Cools the blood, Drain damp, Invigorates blood, Parasites, Resolve phlegm, Smoothes liver qi, Spleen qi)

Neem C (Clear heat, Drain damp, Parasites, Other: Contraceptive)

Soy C (Clear heat, Drain damp, Invigorate blood, Nourish yin, Spleen qi)

St. John's Wort C (Astringe, Bi Syndrome, Clear heat, Smooth liver qi, Stop cough)

Watermelon Seed Cold (Clear heat, drain damp)

Cool the Blood

Centella Cold (Astringe, Clear heat, Drain damp, Cools the blood)

Lime Blossom C (Astringe, Calm the shen, Clear heat/summer heat, Cools the blood, Drain damp, Invigorates blood, Parasites, Resolve phlegm, Smoothes liver qi, Spleen qi)

Drain Damp

Black Currant Seed W? (Drain damp, Spleen Qi, Stop cough)
Camelia Seed C (Drain damp, Spleen qi)
Carrot N (Drain damp, Parasites, Resolve phlegm, Spleen qi)
Centella Cold (Astringe, Clear heat, Drain damp, Cools the blood)
Chamomille C (Calm the shen, Clear heat, Dry damp, Subdue wind)
Cocoa Butter (Calms the shen, Drains damp)
Coffee, Green W (Drain damp, Nourish blood, Tonify yang/heart)
Coffee, Roasted W (Drain damp, Tonify yang/heart)
Copaiba (Drain damp)
Corn N (Drain damp, Nourish yin/heart/kidney, Spleen qi)
Cranberry Seed C (Clear heat, Drain damp)
Grapeseed C (Drain damp, Nourish yin, Tonify qi)
Jojoba (Drain damp, Resolve phlegm)
Lime Blossom C (Astringe, Calm the shen, Clear heat/summer heat, Cools the blood, Drain damp, Invigorates blood, Parasites, Resolve phlegm, Smoothes liver qi, Spleen qi)
Marula C (Drain damp, Nourish yin, Spleen qi)
Monoi N? (Drain damp, Nourish yin/heart, Subdue wind)
Mustard Seed W (Drain damp, Regulate qi, Resolve phlegm/lung, Spleen qi)
Neem C (Clear heat, Drain damp, Parasites, Other: Contraceptive)
Olive (Drain damp, Nourish blood)
Papaya N (Drain damp, Smooth liver qi, Spleen qi)
Pomace Olive (Drain damp, Nourish blood)
Pumpkin Seed N (Drain damp, Parasites, Spleen qi)
Rose Hip W (Astringe, Drain damp, Tonify qi/kidney)
Soy C (Clear heat, Drain damp, Invigorate blood, Nourish yin, Spleen qi)
Watermelon Seed Cold (Clear heat, drain damp)

Food Stagnation

Calendula C (Astringe, Food stagnation, Invigorate blood, Release exterior, Other: Promote mestruation)
Perilla Seed W (Food stasis, Stop cough, Other: Moistens intestine to move bowel)

Invigorate Blood

Andiroba C (Nourish yin, Move qi and blood, Parasites, Spleen qi, Stop cough)

Argan (Invigorate blood, Nourish yin?, Wei qi)

Arnica C? (Move qi and blood)

Babassu Palm C? (Astringe?, Move qi and blood?)

Calendula C (Astringe, Food stagnation, Invigorate blood, Release exterior, Other: Promote menstruation)

Cottonseed (Invigorate blood/lower, Tonify yang, Other: Induces abortion)

Emu C (Move qi and blood, Nourish blood, Nourish yin)

Karanja W (Bi syndrome, Invigorate blood, Nourish blood, Parasites)

Lime Blossom C (Astringe, Calm the shen, Clear heat/summer heat, Cools the blood, Drain damp, Invigorates blood, Parasites, Resolve phlegm, Smoothes liver qi, Spleen qi)

Linseed (flax seed) N (Move qi and blood, Resolve phlegm, Spleen qi)

Meadowfoam (Move blood)

Passion Flower (Calm the shen, Move qi and blood)

Peach Kernel C (Moves qi and blood, Other: Drain abcess, Moisten intestine to move bowel)

Poppy Seed N (Move qi and blood/chest, Other: Contain lung qi, Bind large intestine)

Safflower W (Invigorate blood, Other: Promote menstruation)

Sea Buckthorn (Move qi and blood, Nourish yin)

Shea Butter (Move qi and blood?, Resolve phlegm)

Soy C (Clear heat, Drain damp, Invigorate blood, Nourish yin, Spleen qi)

Tamanu C (Move qi and blood)

Wheatgerm C (Calm the shen, Invigorate blood, Nourish yin)

Witch Hazel (Astringe, Calm the shen, Invigorate blood, Spleen qi, Tonify qi)

Nourish Blood

Avocado C (Nourish blood, Nourish yin, Smoothes liver qi)

Black Raspberry Seed N (Astringe, Nourish blood, Nourish yin/kidney/liver)

Blackberry Seed N (Astringe, Nourish blood, Nourish yin/kidney, Spleen qi)

Borage C (Nourish blood, Nourish liver yin, Smooth liver qi)

Coffee, Green W (Drain damp, Nourish blood, Tonify yang/heart)

Cohune Nut (Nourish blood?, Nourish yin?)

Egg N (Nourish blood, Nourish yin, Spleen qi, Tonify qi)

Emu C (Move qi and blood, Nourish blood, Nourish yin)

Evening Primrose (Nourish blood, Nourish liver yin, Spleen qi)

Karanja W (Bi syndrome, Invigorate blood, Nourish blood, Parasites)

Moringa (Nourish blood, Nourish yin)

Olive (Drain damp, Nourish blood)

Pomace Olive (Drain damp, Nourish blood)

Red Raspberry Seed N (Astringe, Nourish blood, Nourish yin/kidney/liver)

Sesame (Nourish blood, Nourish yin/Jing essence, Parasites)

Nourish Yin

Acai Oil (Nourish yin, Tonify qi)

Almond N (sweet) N (Nourish yin/lung, Release the exterior, Resolve phlegm, Stop cough, Tonify qi/lung, Other: Regulates colon)

Aloe Cold (Clear heat/liver fire, Nourish yin, Parasites, Other: Purges downward, Constipation)

Andiroba C (Nourish yin, Move qi and blood, Parasites, Spleen qi, Stop cough)

Argan (Invigorate blood, Nourish yin?, Wei qi)

Avocado C (Nourish blood, Nourish yin, Smoothes liver qi)

Baobab (Nourish yin)

Black Cumin Seed (Nourish yin, Spleen qi, Tonify qi)

Black Raspberry Seed N (Astringe, Nourish blood, Nourish yin/kidney/liver)

Blackberry Seed N (Astringe, Nourish blood, Nourish yin/kidney, Spleen qi)

Borage C (Nourish blood, Nourish liver yin, Smooth liver qi)

Castor (Nourish yin, Parasites, Other: Purge Colon in constipation)

Coconut W (Nourish yin/heart, Subdue wind)

Cohune Nut (Nourish blood?, Nourish yin?)

Corn N (Drain damp, Nourish yin/heart/kidney, Spleen qi)

Cucumber Seed C (Clear heat/summerheat, Nourish yin, Parasites, Spleen qi)

Egg N (Nourish blood, Nourish yin, Spleen qi, Tonify qi)

Emu C (Move qi and blood, Nourish blood, Nourish yin)

Evening Primrose (Nourish blood, Nourish liver yin, Spleen qi)

Grapeseed C (Drain damp, Nourish yin, Tonify qi)

Hemp Seed N (Nourish yin)

Kukui Nut C (Nourish yin)

Macadamia (Nourish yin)

Manketti (Nourish yin, Tonify qi)

Mango Seed W (Nourish yin, Spleen qi)

Marula C (Drain damp, Nourish yin, Spleen qi)

Monoi N? (Drain damp, Nourish yin/heart, Subdue wind)

Moringa (Nourish blood, Nourish yin)

Oat W (Nourish yin, Regulate qi, Spleen qi, Tonify qi)

Palm Kernal W (Nourish yin/heart, Subdue wind)

Peanut W (Astringe, Nourish yin/lung, Spleen qi, Stop cough)

Pistachio N (Nourish yin, Tonify qi)

Plum Kernel C (Nourish yin/liver)

Red Raspberry Seed N (Astringe, Nourish blood, Nourish yin/kidney/liver)

Sea Buckthorn (Move qi and blood, Nourish yin)
Sesame (Nourish blood, Nourish yin/Jing essence, Parasites)
Soy C (Clear heat, Drain damp, Invigorate blood, Nourish yin, Spleen qi)
Wheatgerm C (Calm the shen, Invigorate blood, Nourish yin)

Parasites

Aloe Cold (Clear heat/liver fire, Nourish yin, Parasites, Other: Purges downward, Constipation)
Andiroba C (Nourish yin, Move qi and blood, Parasites, Spleen qi, Stop cough)
Carrot N (Drain damp, Parasites, Resolve phlegm, Spleen qi)
Castor (Nourish yin, Parasites, Other: Purge Colon in constipation)
Cucumber Seed C (Clear heat/summerheat, Nourish yin, Parasites, Spleen qi)
Karanja W (Bi syndrome, Invigorate blood, Nourish blood, Parasites)
Lime Blossom C (Astringe, Calm the shen, Clear heat/summer heat, Cools the blood, Drain damp, Invigorates blood, Parasites, Resolve phlegm, Smoothes liver qi, Spleen qi)
Neem C (Clear heat, Drain damp, Parasites, Other: Contraceptive)
Pomegranite Seed C (Parasites)
Pumpkin Seed N (Drain damp, Parasites, Spleen qi)
Sesame (Nourish blood, Nourish yin/Jing essence, Parasites)

Regulate Qi

Andiroba C (Nourish yin, Move qi and blood, Parasites, Spleen qi, Stop cough)

Arnica C? (Move qi and blood)

Babassu Palm C? (Astringe?, Move qi and blood?)

Cumin Seed W (Regulate qi, Spleen qi)

Emu C (Move qi and blood, Nourish blood, Nourish yin)

Linseed (Flax Seed) N (Move qi and blood, Resolve phlegm, Spleen qi)

Mustard Seed W (Drain damp, Regulate qi, Resolve phlegm/lung, Spleen qi)

Oat W (Nourish yin, Regulate qi, Spleen qi, Tonify qi)

Passion Flower (Calm the shen, Move qi and blood)

Peach Kernel C (Moves qi and blood, Other: Drain abcess, Moisten intestine to move bowel)

Poppy Seed N (Move qi and blood/chest, Other: Contain lung qi, Bind large intestine)

Rapeseed W (Regulate qi, Resolve phlegm)

Sea Buckthorn (Move qi and blood, Nourish yin)

Shea Butter (Move qi and blood?, Resolve phlegm)

Tamanu C (Move qi and blood)

Release the Exterior

Almond (sweet) N (Nourish yin/lung, Release the exterior, Resolve phlegm, Stop cough, Tonify qi/lung, Other: Regulates colon)

Calendula C (Astringe, Food stagnation, Invigorate blood, Release exterior, Other: Promote mestruation)

Resolve Phlegm

Almond (sweet) N (Nourish yin/lung, Release the exterior, Resolve phlegm, Stop cough, Tonify qi/lung, Other: Regulates colon)

Carrot N (Drain damp, Parasites, Resolve phlegm, Spleen qi)

Jojoba (Drain damp, Resolve phlegm)

Lime Blossom C (Astringe, Calm the shen, Clear heat/summer heat, Cools the blood, Drain damp, Invigorates blood, Parasites, Resolve phlegm, Smoothes liver qi, Spleen qi)

Linseed (flax seed) N (Move qi and blood, Resolve phlegm, Spleen qi)

Mustard Seed W (Drain damp, Regulate qi, Resolve phlegm/lung, Spleen qi)

Rapeseed W (Regulate qi, Resolve phlegm)

Shea Butter (Move qi and blood?, Resolve phlegm)

Smooth Liver Qi

Avocado C (Nourish blood, Nourish yin, Smooth liver qi)

Borage C (Nourish blood, Nourish liver yin, Smooth liver qi)

Lime Blossom C (Astringe, Calm the shen, Clear heat/summer heat, Cools the blood, Drain damp, Invigorates blood, Parasites, Resolve phlegm, Smoothes liver qi, Spleen qi)

Papaya N (Drain damp, Smooth liver qi, Spleen qi)

St. John's Wort C (Astringe, Bi Syndrome, Clear heat, Smooth liver qi, Stop cough)

Spleen Qi

Andiroba C (Nourish yin, Move qi and blood, Parasites, Spleen qi, Stop cough)

Black Cumin Seed (Nourish yin, Spleen qi, Tonify qi)

Blackberry Seed N (Astringe, Nourish blood, Nourish yin/kidney, Spleen qi)

Black Currant Seed W? (Drain damp, Spleen Qi, Stop cough)

Camelina (Spleen qi, Tonify qi/lung)

Camelia Seed C (Drain damp, Spleen qi)

Carrot N (Drain damp, Parasites, Resolve phlegm, Spleen qi)

Cherry Kernel W (Astringe, Spleen qi, Tonify qi)

Corn N (Drain damp, Nourish yin/heart/kidney, Spleen qi)

Cucumber Seed C (Clear heat/summerheat, Nourish yin, Parasites, Spleen qi)

Cumin Seed W (Regulate qi, Spleen qi)

Egg N (Nourish blood, Nourish yin, Spleen qi, Tonify qi)

Evening Primrose (Nourish blood, Nourish liver yin, Spleen qi)

Hazelnut (Spleen qi, Tonify qi/Yuan qi)

Lime Blossom C (Astringe, Calm the shen, Clear heat/summer heat, Cools the blood, Drain damp, Invigorates blood, Parasites, Resolve phlegm, Smoothes liver qi, Spleen qi)

Linseed (flax seed) N (Move qi and blood, Resolve phlegm, Spleen qi)

Mango Seed W (Nourish yin, Spleen qi)

Marula C (Drain damp, Nourish yin, Spleen qi)

Mustard Seed W (Drain damp, Regulate qi, Resolve phlegm/lung, Spleen qi)

Oat W (Nourish yin, Regulate qi, Spleen qi, Tonify qi)

Papaya N (Drain damp, Smooth liver qi, Spleen qi)

Peanut W (Astringe, Nourish yin/lung, Spleen qi, Stop cough)

Pumpkin Seed N (Drain damp, Parasites, Spleen qi)

Rice Bran W (Spleen qi, Tonify qi)

Soy C (Clear heat, Drain damp, Invigorate blood, Nourish yin, Spleen qi)

Sunflower W (Spleen qi, Tonify qi)

Witch Hazel (Astringe, Calm the shen, Invigorate blood, Spleen qi, Tonify qi)

Stop Cough

Almond (sweet) N (Nourish yin/lung, Release the exterior, Resolve phlegm, Stop cough, Tonify qi/lung, Other: Regulates colon)

Andiroba C (Nourish yin, Move qi and blood, Parasites, Spleen qi, Stop cough)

Apricot Kernel W (Stops cough, Other: Moistens Large Intestine, Purges downward)

Black Currant Seed W? (Drain damp, Spleen Qi, Stop cough)

Peanut W (Astringe, Nourish yin/lung, Spleen qi, Stop cough)

Perilla Seed W (Food stasis, Stop cough, Other: Moistens intestine to move bowel)

St. John's Wort C (Astringe, Bi Syndrome, Clear heat, Smooth liver qi, Stop cough)

Subdue Wind

Chamomille C (Calm the shen, Clear heat, Dry damp, Subdue wind)

Coconut W (Nourish yin/heart, Subdue wind)

Monoi N? (Drain damp, Nourish yin/heart, Subdue wind)

Palm Kernal W (Nourish yin/heart, Subdue wind)

Tonify Qi

Acai Oil (Nourish yin, Tonify qi)
Almond (sweet) N (Nourish yin/lung, Release the exterior, Resolve phlegm, Stop cough, Tonify qi/lung, Other: Regulates colon)
Black Cumin Seed (Nourish yin, Spleen qi, Tonify qi)
Camelina (Spleen qi, Tonify qi/lung)
Cherry Kernel W (Astringe, Spleen qi, Tonify qi)
Egg N (Nourish blood, Nourish yin, Spleen qi, Tonify qi)
Grapeseed C (Drain damp, Nourish yin, Tonify qi)
Hazelnut (Spleen qi, Tonify qi/Yuan qi)
Manketti (Nourish yin, Tonify qi)
Oat W (Nourish yin, Regulate qi, Spleen qi, Tonify qi)
Pistachio N (Nourish yin, Tonify qi)
Rice Bran W (Spleen qi, Tonify qi)
Rose Hip W (Astringe, Drain damp, Tonify qi/kidney)
Sisymbrium (Tonify qi)
Sunflower W (Spleen qi, Tonify qi)
Witch Hazel (Astringe, Calm the shen, Invigorate blood, Spleen qi, Tonify qi)

Tonify Yang

Coffee, Green W (Drain damp, Nourish blood, Tonify yang/heart)
Coffee, Roasted W (Drain damp, Tonify yang/heart)
Cottonseed (Invigorate blood/lower, Tonify yang, Other: Induces abortion)
Walnut W (Tonify yang/kidney, Other: Helps kidneys grasp qi.)

Wei Qi

Argan (Invigorate blood, Nourish yin?, Wei qi)
Pecan (Wei qi)

Other

Almond (bitter) (Diffuses, Disperses lung qi)
Pequi
Pracaxi
Yangu

Essential Oils
Alphabetical List

Symbolic Key

T: Top note
M: Middle note
B: Base note

C: Cooling
W: Warming

s: slightly, as in "slightly cooling."
d: drying, as in "warming and drying."

Notes

-Some oils can be used as more than one note. For instance, Peppermint can be used as either a top or middle note. Ginger can be used as a middle or base note.

-Some oils are listed as "hot" or "cold." These oils are particularly warming or cooling, so we specified that.

-Some oils have meridian tropism. See **Jeffrey Yuen's** Materia Medica for more specifics on that. We indicate if certain oils have tropism with reference to its functions. For instance, Cypress will clear heat, but has an affinity for the lung. So we list it as "clear heat/lung." There are many oils that tonify qi of a specific organ/meridian system. Consider them all to be general qi tonics, but with special tropism for those organ/meridian systems.

Essential Oils: Alphabetical

Angelica BW (Calm the shen, Invigorate blood, Nourish blood, Smooth liver qi, Spleen qi, Tonify qi/lung, Wei qi, Other: Ease cough, Expel phlegm, Open the diaphragm) Apiaceae/Umbelliferae
Cautions: Photosensitive, Pregnancy, Diabetes

Anise MC (Clear heat, Food stagnation, Regulate qi, Smooth liver qi, Stop cough, Other: Promote lactation) Apiaceae/Umbelliferae
Cautions: Mild estrogenic, Yin deficiency, Cancer, Pregnancy

Ajowan Seed TW (Parasites, Spleen qi, Tonifies Qi/Lung, Tonify Yang, Wei qi)
Cautions: Pregnancy

Atlas Cedar BC (Open orifice, Resolve phlegm, Smooth liver qi) Coniferae
Cautions: Prepubescent children, Pregnancy

Balsam of Peru BW (Calm the Shen, Moves qi and blood, Parasites, Resolve phlegm, Tonifies Qi/Heart, Wei qi) Fabaceae
Cautions: May cause sensitization, Pregnancy, Breastfeeding

Basil T/MW (Food stasis, Nourish yin/liver, Release the exterior, Spleen qi, Tonify qi//kidney, Tonify yang, Wei qi, Other: Promote lactation, Relieve uterine contraction) Lamiaceae/Labiatae
Cautions: Use in small doses, Pregnancy

Bay Laurel TsC (Food stasis, Regulate qi/stomach, Resolve hot phlegm) Lauraceae
Cautions: Narcotic in large doses, Pregnancy

Benzoin BW (Bi/expel damp cold, Drain damp/lower, Spleen qi, Stop coughing, Tonify yang/spleen, Other: Diffuse lung qi) Styracaceae
Cautions: Heat, Empty heat

Bergamot T/MsC (Clear heat/fire toxin, Drain damp, Food stagnation, Regulate qi, Release exterior, Smooth liver qi, Wei qi) Rutacae
Cautions: Photosensitive

Birch MW (Bi/expel wind damp cold, Clear Heat, Drain damp, Release exterior, Other: Open joints) Betulaceae
Cautions: Kidney toxicity, Kidney deficiency, May thin the blood, Pregnancy, Breastfeeding

Bitter Orange TCold (Food stagnation, Regulate qi/liver/stomach, Spleen qi, Smooth liver qi) Rutacae
Cautions: Photosensitive, Qi deficiency, Cold stomach

Black Pepper MHot (Release exterior, Spleen qi, Tonify qi/kidney, Tonify yang, Wei qi) Piperacea
Cautions: Deficiency heat, Pregnancy

Blue Yarrow TC (Clear Heat, Moves qi and blood, Tonifies qi/heart)
Cautions: Pregnancy

Cajeput MC (Bi/Expel damp hot, Drain damp/lower jiao, Move qi and blood, Parasites, Release exterior, Tonify qi/lung) Myrtaceae

Camphor THot (Bi/expel wind damp, Invigorate blood, Open orifice, Parasites, Resolve phlegm) Lauraceae
Cautions: Pregnancy, Epilepsy, Can irritate mucous membranes, Toxicity

Caraway MW (Resolve damp phlegm, Spleen qi, Tonify qi, Other: Descend qi) Apiaceae/Umbelliferae
Cautions: Pregnancy, Children under 3, Cancer

Cardamom MW (Food stasis, Invigorate blood, Regulate qi, Spleen qi, Stop coughing, Tonify qi/Lung) Zingiberaceae
Cautions: Yin deficiency, Blood deficiency

Carrot (seed) MC (Drain damp, Nourish blood, Nourish yin/liver, Smooth liver qi) Apiaceae/Umbelliferae

Cedarwood BC (Clear heat/Lung, Dry damp/lower, Spleen qi, Tonify qi/lung, Tonify yang/kidney/spleen, Other: Relieve itch) Cupressaceae
Cautions: Pregnancy, Prepubescent children

Celery Seed MC (Bi/wind damp, Clear fire toxin, Drain damp, Food stasis, Nourish yin/liver, Regulate qi, Smooth liver qi, Spleen qi, Tonify qi/kidney) Apiaceae/Umbelliferae
Cautions: Estrogenic, Photosensitive, Pregnancy, Breastfeeding

Cinnamon BHot (Astringe/blood, Bi/expel wind damp, Drain damp, Invigorate blood, Nourish blood, Parasites, Spleen qi, Tonify qi, Tonify yang, Warm interior to expel cold, Wei qi, Other: Regulate menstruation) Lauraceae
Cautions: Heat/empty heat, Mucous membranes, Pregnancy, May sensitize skin, Kidney, Liver toxicity, May prevent coagulation

Cinnamon Leaf MW (Invigorate blood, Release exterior, Spleen qi, Other: Promote sweating, Stimulate childbirth) Lauraceae
Cautions: Heat/empty heat

Cistus BsW (Smooth liver qi, Tonify spleen, Other: Stop bleeding) Cistaceae
Cautions: Pregnancy

Citronella TCold (Release the exterior, Tonify qi, Wei qi) Graminae
Cautions: Yang deficiency

Clary Sage MC (Clear heat/stomach, Cool the blood, Nourish yin, Smooth liver qi, Spleen qi, Subdue wind, Tonify qi/heart/lung, Other: Clear empty heat, Encourages labor, Regulates menses, Running piglet qi) Lamiaceae/Labiatae
Cautions: Estrogenic, Can be narcotic in larger doses, Cancer, Pregancy, Alcohol consumption

Clove THot (Parasites, Spleen qi, Tonify yang/kidney, Warm interior to expel cold) Myrtaceae
Cautions: Yin deficiency, Pregnancy, May prevent coagulation

Coriander MW (Bi/expel wind damp cold, Nourish yin/liver, Spleen qi, Tonify qi/kidney, Wei qi) Apiaceae/Umbelliferae
Cautions: Pregnancy, Can be photosensitive

Cumin MsW (Invigorate blood, Smooth liver qi, Spleen qi, Tonify qi/heart) Apiaceae/Umbelliferae
Cautions: Photosensitive, Pregnancy

Cypress MBsC (Astringe, Clear heat/lung, Move qi and blood, Stop coughing, Other: Ascend spleen qi, Assist kidney to grasp lung qi) Cupressaceae
Cautions: Hypertension, Cancer

Dill BW (Drain damp, Food stasis, Invigorate blood, Spleen qi, Stop coughing, Other: Lactation, Promote bile secretion) Apiaceae/Umbelliferae
Cautions: Heat/empty heat, Yin deficiency, Liver wind/ascending yang, Pregnancy

Elemi BWd (Invigorate blood/chest, Regulate qi/chest, Resolve phlegm) Berseraceae
Cautions: Pregnancy

Eucalyptus Citriodora TC (Drain damp, Move qi and blood, Wei qi,) Myrtaceae
Cautions: Children

Eucalyptus Globulus T/MW (Drain damp, Move qi and blood, Parasites, Release the exterior, Wei qi) Myrtaceae
Cautions: Children and babies

Eucalyptus Radiata TW (Drain damp, Resolve Phlegm, Tonify qi, Wei qi) Myrtaceae

Eucalyptus Smithii TC (Drain damp, Resolve Phlegm, Tonifies Qi, Wei qi) Myrtaceae
Cautions: Children 3 and under, Pregnancy

Fennel MW (Drain damp, Nourish yin, Spleen qi, Tonify qi/lung, Tonify yang) Apiaceae/Umbelliferae
Cautions: Estrogenic, Heat, Interior wind, Pregnancy, Cancer, Hypothyroidism

Fir MC (Bi/expel damp hot, Clear heat, Dry damp/lower, Resolve phlegm/damp, Stop coughing, Tonify qi/lung, Other: Help kidneys grasp qi) Pinaceae

Frankincense BsCd (Calm the shen, Clear heat/Lung/Stomach, Dry damp, Nourish blood/liver, Resolve phlegm, Strongly move qi and blood, Tonify qi/lung, Other: Reduce swelling) Berceraceae
Cautions: Pregnancy

Galbanum M/BC (Bi/expel damp hot, Calm the shen, Smooth liver qi, Tonify qi/lung,) Apiaceae/Umbelliferae

Garlic MW (Parasites, Other: Detoxify) Liliaceae, Amaryllidaceae
Cautions: Heat/empty heat, Yin deficiency

Geranium T/MN (Astringe/lower, Calm the shen, Cool the blood, Food stasis, Nourish yin, Parasites, Smooth liver qi, Spleen qi, Tonify qi/kidney, Other: Regulates menses) Gereniaceae
Cautions: Estrogenic, Pregnancy

German Chamomile MC (Calm the shen, Clear heat/liver/stomach/heart, Drain Damp, Nourish yin/heart, Smoothes Liver Qi, Spleen qi, Subdue wind, Tonify qi/Lung) Asteraceae/Compositae

Ginger M/BHot (Invigorate blood, Parasites, Release exterior, Spleen qi, Tonify qi/lung/heart/kidney, Tonify yang, Warm interior to expel cold, Wei qi, Other: Harmonize blends) Zingiberaceae
Cautions: Heat/empty heat, Stomach fire

Grapefruit TsWd (Drain damp, Food stasis, Regulate qi, Resolve phlegm, Smooth liver qi, Other: Promote bile production) Rutaceae
Cautions: Photosensitive, Heat patterns

Helichrysum BC (Bi/expel damp hot, Clear heat/Lung/Liver/Fire Toxin, Cool the blood, Move qi and blood, Nourish blood, Smooth liver qi, Wei qi) Asteracea/Compositae
Cautions: Yang deficiency

Ho Leaf MC (Release exterior, Resolve phlegm, Spleen qi, Other: armonize Blends) Lauraceae
Cautions: Yang deficiency

Hyssop MW(Bi/expel damp cold, Invigorate blood, Spleen qi, Tonify qi/lung/heart, Tonify yang) Lamiaceae/Labiatae
Cautions: Neurotoxic, Liver wind, Glaucoma, Cancer, Pregnancy, Children, Excessive use can cause asthma, seizures, hypertension.

Hyssop Linalool MC (Clear heat/lung) Lamiaceae/Labiatae
Cautions: Yang deficiency, Ragweed allergy

Inula BsC (Clear heat/Lung, Drain/transform damp/upper, Stop coughing, Tonify qi/heart, Wei qi) Asteracea/Compositae
Cautions: Toxicity

Jasmine BC (Clear heat/Liver, Nourish yin, Other: Clear empty heat, Promote childbirth) Oleaceae
Cautions: Yang deficiency

Juniper MW (Drain damp, Invigorate blood, Resolve phlegm, Spleen qi, Tonify yang/strongly, Other: Promote menstruation) Cupressaceae
Cautions: Kidney yin deficiency, Kidney toxicity, Pregnancy

Lavender T/MC (Calm the Shen, Clear heat/lung/liver, Nourish yin, Parasites, Regulate qi, Release the exterior, Smooth liver qi, Tonify qi/heart, Tonify yang/heart, Other: Diffuse lung qi) Lamiaceae/Labiatae

Lavendin MC (Clear heat/lung/liver, Smooth liver qi) Lamiaceae/Labiatae
Cautions: Yang deficiency, (Not toxic when diluted.)

Lemon TCd (Bi/damp Invigorate blood, Clear heat/liver/GB/stomach, Spleen qi, Wei qi, Other: Break up stones) Rutaceae
Cautions: Photosensitive

Lemon Verbena TC (Clear heat/Heart/Liver, Smooth liver qi) Lamiaceae/Labiatae
Cautions: Mildly photosensitive

Lemongrass TW (Nourish blood, Spleen qi, Tonify yang, Warm interior to expel cold, Wei qi) Graminae
Cautions: Heat/empty heat, Glaucoma, Children, Prostatic hyperplasia, Slight risk of sensitization

Lime TC (Regulate qi/stomach/spleen, Wei qi, Other: Uplift mood) Rutaceae
Cautions: Photosensitive

Litsea MW (Bi/expel wind damp cold, Invigorate blood/lower, Regulate qi/lower, Release the exterior, Spleen qi, Tonify yang) Lauraceae
Cautions: Yin deficiency with heat

Lovage BCold (Clear heat/stomach/kidney, Drain damp, Resolve phlegm, spleen qi) Apiaceae/Umbelliferae
Cautions: Photosensitive, Toxic

Mandarin TC (Calm the Shen, Food stasis, Regulate qi, Spleen qi, Subdue wind) Rutaceae

Marigold BC (Clear heat, Resolve hot phlegm, Other: Promote bile secretion) Asteracea/Compositae
Cautions: Photosensitive, Toxic, Epilepsy, Pregnancy

Melissa MC (Astringe/blood, Clear heat/liver/heart/wei, Cools the blood, Food stasis, Parasites, Regulate qi, Release the exterior, Smooth liver qi, Other: Open and relax the chest) Lamiaceae/Labiatae
Cautions: Can be sensitizing in high doses.

Mimosa MCold (Calm the shen, Clear heat/fire toxin, Cool the blood) Mimosaceae
Cautions: Cold or Deficient yang

Mugwort M/BW (Warm interior to expel cold, Other: Warm the uterus to promote menstruation) Asteraceae
Cautions: Heat/empty heat, Pregnancy, Neurotoxic

Myrrh BC (Clear heat/Lung/Stomach, Dry damp, Move qi and blood, Spleen qi, Other: Promotes healing of wounds) Burseraceae
Cautions: Pregnancy, Uterine bleeding

Myrtle M/BCd (Astringe, Clear heat/Lung, Drain damp/lower, Smooth liver qi, Wei qi) Myrtaceae
Cautions: Yang deficiency, Cold

Narcissus BC (Calm the Shen, Other: Harmonize kidneys and heart) Amaryllidaceae
Cautions: Yang deficiency, Cold

Neroli M/BC (Clear heat/Heart/fire toxin, Spleen qi, Tonify qi) Rutaceae

Niaouli MC (Bi/wind damp/lower, Invigorate blood, Parasites, Release the exterior, Spleen qi, Tonify qi/lung/kidney, Wei qi) Myrtaceae
Cautions: Pregnancy, Children

Nutmeg MW (Nourish blood, Move qi and blood, Spleen qi, Tonify yang/spleen/kidney, Warm interior to expel cold) Myristicaceae
Cautions: Diarrhea due to heat, Liver wind/Ascending yang, Epilepsy, Liver toxicity, Pregnancy, High doses can produce delirium, convulsions, Hallucinations, Dizziness, Fainting, Cancer

Oakmoss BC (Nourish yin/lung, Resolve phlegm) Usneaceae
Caution: Can be sensitizing, Epilepsy, Toxicity, Pregnancy

Onion MW (Invigorate blood, Parasites, Resolve phlegm, Warm interior to expel cold) Liliaceae
Cautions: Heat/empty heat

Orange TC (Clear heat/Heart, Food stasis, Regulate qi, Release exterior, Smooth liver qi, Spleen qi, Other: Clear heart fire) Rutaceae
Caution: Photosensitive

Oregano MW (Bi/expel wind damp cold, Move qi and blood, Open orifice, Parasites, Spleen qi, Wei qi, Other: Promotes menstruation) Lamiaceae/Labiatae
Cautions: Heat/empty heat, Pregnancy, Liver toxicity

Palmarosa TC (Clear heat, Drain damp/lower, Nourish yin, Release the exterior, Smooth liver qi, Other: Clear damp heat skin outbreaks) Poaceae
Parsley MW (Drain damp/lower, Invigorate blood, Regulate qi/stomach, Other: Abortion, Childbirth, Promote menstruation) Umbelliferae
Cautions: Neurotoxic, Liver toxic, Pregnancy, Breastfeeding

Patchouli BsW (Clear summer heat, Release the exterior, Strongly tonify spleen qi, Other: Release suppressed emotion) Lamiaceae/Labiatae

Pennyroyal T/MW (Food stasis, Spleen qi, Stop coughing, Other: Promote bile, Regulate menses) Lamiaceae/Labiatae
Cautions: Pregnancy

Peppermint T/MC (Clear heat, Open portals, Regulate qi, Release exterior, Smooth liver qi, Spleen qi, Tonify qi/lung, Other: Move wei qi, Relieve itch) Lamiaceae/Labiatae
Cautions: Young children, Cardiac fibrillation, Epilepsy, Mucous membranes, Neurotoxic

Petitgrain T/MC (Calm the shen, Drain damp, Regulate qi/chest, Smooth liver qi) Rutaceae

Pine MW (Release the exterior, Resolve phlegm, Spleen qi, Stop cough, Tonify qi/lung/kidney, Tonify yang, Other: Descend qi to kidneys) Pinaceae
Cautions: Yin deficiency, Blood deficiency

Ravensare MC (Clear heat/lung, Release exterior) Lauraceae

Roman Chamomille MC (Calm the Shen, Clear heat/liver, Nourish blood, Nourish yin/liver, Regulate qi, Smooth liver qi, Subdue wind) Asteraceae/Compositae
Cautions: Yang deficiency, Ragweed allergy

Rosalina TC (Clear heat/stomach, Release the exterior) Myrtaceae
Caution: Pregnancy

Rose BN (Clear heat/liver, Cool the blood, Invigorate blood, Nourish yin, Open orifice, Smooth liver qi, Other: Harmonize kidney/heart, Promote bile) Roseaceae

Rosemary T/MW (Nourish blood, Regulate qi, Release the exterior, Spleen qi, Tonify qi/kidney/heart, Tonify yang, Warm the interior to expel cold) Lamiaceae/Labiatae
Cautions: Heat/empty heat, Pregnancy, Children, Rebellious qi, Hypertension

Rosewood MN (Parasites, Regulate qi, Release the exterior, Smooth liver qi, Spleen qi, Tonify qi, Wei qi) Lauraceae

Sage T/MC (Clear heat/stomach, Nourish yin, Release exterior, Resolve phlegm, Tonifies Qi/kidney, Other: Promote bile, Wei qi) Lamiaceae/Labiatae
Cautions: May be estrogenic, Seizures, Pregnancy, Tisserand recommends avoiding Sage in aromatherapy.

Sandalwood BsC (Calm the Shen, Clear heat/Lower Jiao, Dry damp, Nourish yin, Moves qi and blood, Other: Opens diaphragm) Santalaceae

Sassafras BHot (Bi/expel wind damp cold, Invigorate blood, Other: Promote menstruation) Lauraceae
Cautions: Very Dangerous, Toxicity, Pregnancy, Cancer

Savory MW (Nourish blood, Parasites, Resolve phlegm, Spleen qi, Tonify qi) Lamiaceae/Labiatae
Cautions: Heat/empty heat, Pregnancy

Spearmint T/MC (Calm the shen, Release the exterior, Smooth liver qi, Spleen qi, Wei qi, Other: Relieve itch) Lamiaceae/Labiatae
Cautions: Neurotoxic, Pregnancy, Mucous membranes

Spikenard BC (Calms the shen, Clear heat/Heart, Nourish yin/heart, Smooth liver qi, Subdue wind) Valerianaceae
Cautions: Exogenous conditions

Spruce T/MW (Bi/expel wind cold, Calm the shen, Stop coughing, Tonify qi, Tonify yang, Wei qi, Other: Helps kidneys graps lung qi) Pinaceae
Caution: May irritate the skin

Styrax BW (Bi/expel wind damp cold, Food stasis, Invigorate blood, Open portals, Parasites, Resolve phlegm/turbid, Other: Promote menstruation) Styracaceae
Cautions: Pregnancy, Yang collapse, High fever

Sweet Marjoram T/MC (Bi/expel damp hot, Clear heat/liver, Food stasis, Regulate qi, Release exterior, Smooth liver qi, Stop coughing) Lamiaceae/Labiatae
Cautions: Asthma, Pregnancy

Tangerine TC (Nourish blood, Move qi and blood, Spleen qi) Rutaceae
Cautions: May be photosensitive

Tarragon MW (Food stasis, Moves qi and blood, Nourish Blood, Parasites, Spleen qi, Tonify Qi/heart, Other: Promote menstruation) Asteraceae
Cautions: Pregnancy, Cancer

Tea Tree MC (Clear heat, Dry damp, Invigorate blood, Parasites, Release exterior, Tonify qi, Wei qi) Myraceae

Terebinth MW (Bi/expel wind damp cold, Release Exterior, Subdue wind) Pinaceae
Cautions: Yin deficiency/liver/kidney, Blood deficiency, Epilepsy

Thuja MW (Bi/expel damp cold/lower) Cupressaceae
Cautions: Neurotoxic, Pregnancy

Thyme Geraniol MC (Nourish blood)
Cautions: Hypertension, May irritate skin, Mucous membranes

Thyme Linalool MC (Clear heat/lung/stomach, Parasites, Tonify qi) Lamiaceae/Labiatae
Cautions: Glaucoma

Valerian BW (Nourish blood, Nourishes yin, Parasites, Regulate Qi, Subdue wind, Tonifies Qi/heart, Tonify Yang/heart, Wei qi) Valerianaceae
Cautions: Qi deficiency, Yang deficiency, Pregnancy, Children

Vanilla BsW (Calm the Shen, Tonify qi/kidney, Other: Release suppressed emotion) Orchidaceae

Vetiver BC (Calm the Shen, Clear heat, Cool the blood, Invigorate blood, Nourish blood, Nourish yin, Smooth liver qi, Spleen qi, Tonify qi/heart) Gramineae

Violet BC (Calm the Shen, Clear heat/lung/fire toxin, Tonify qi/lung/heart, Other: Harmonize heart and kidney) Violaceae
Cautions: Yang deficiency, Cold

Wintergreen MW (Bi/expel wind damp hot, Release the exterior, Smooth liver qi) Ericaceae
Cautions: Kidney toxicity in overuse, Pregnancy

Yarrow MCold (Clear heat, Moves qi and blood, Smoothes liver qi, Spleen qi, Tonifies qi/heart/kidney, Other: Ascend spleen qi, Promote sweating) Asteracea/Compositae
Cautions: Neurotoxic, Children, Pregnancy, Ragweed allergy

Ylang Ylang MBC (Calm the Shen, Clear heat/heart fire, Cool the blood, Nourish yin/heart/kidney, Tonifies qi/kidney, Wei qi) Annonaceae
Cautions: Yang deficiency, Cold

Essential Oils
Materia Medica

Symbolic Key

T: Top note
M: Middle note
B: Base note

C: Cooling
W: Warming

s: slightly, as in "slightly cooling."
d: drying, as in "warming and drying."

Notes

-Some oils can be used as more than one note. For instance, Peppermint can be used as either a top or middle note. Ginger can be used as a middle or base note.

-Some oils are listed as "hot" or "cold." These oils are particularly warming or cooling, so we specified that.

-Some oils have meridian tropism. See Jeffrey Yuen's Materia Medica for more specifics on that. We indicate if certain oils have tropism with reference to its functions. For instance, Cypress will clear heat, but has an affinity for the lung. So we list it as "clear heat/lung." There are many oils that tonify qi of specific organ/meridian system. Consider them all to be general qi tonics, but with special tropism for those organ/meridian systems.

ASTRINGE

Top Neutral...
Geranium T/MN (Astringe/lower, Calm the shen, Cool the blood, Food stasis, Nourish yin, Parasites, Smooth liver qi, Spleen qi, Tonify qi/kidney, Other: Regulates menses) Gereniaceae
Cautions: Estrogenic, Pregnancy
Middle Neutral...
Geranium T/MN (Astringe/lower, Calm the shen, Cool the blood, Food stasis, Nourish yin, Parasites, Smooth liver qi, Spleen qi, Tonify qi/kidney, Other: Regulates menses) Gereniaceae
Cautions: Estrogenic, Pregnancy
Middle Cooling..
Cypress M/BsC (Astringe, Clear heat/lung, Move qi and blood, Stop coughing, Other: Ascend spleen qi, Assist kidney to grasp lung qi) Cupressaceae
Cautions: Hypertension, Cancer
Melissa MC (Astringe/blood, Clear heat/liver/heart/wei, Cools the blood, Food stasis, Parasites, Regulate qi, Release the exterior, Smooth liver qi, Other: Open and relax the chest) Lamiaceae/Labiatae
Cautions: Can be sensitizing in high doses.
Myrtle M/BCd (Astringe, Clear heat/Lung, Drain damp/lower, Smooth liver qi, Wei qi) Myrtaceae
Cautions: Yang deficiency, Cold
Base Warming..
Cinnamon BHot (Astringe/blood, Bi/expel wind damp, Drain damp, Invigorate blood, Nourish blood, Parasites, Spleen qi, Tonify qi, Tonify yang, Warm interior to expel cold, Wei qi, Other: Regulate menstruation) Lauraceae
Cautions: Heat/empty heat, Mucous membranes, Pregnancy, May sensitize skin, Kidney, Liver toxicity, May prevent coagulation
Base Cooling...
Cypress M/BsC (Astringe, Clear heat/lung, Move qi and blood, Stop coughing, Other: Ascend spleen qi, Assist kidney to grasp lung qi) Cupressaceae
Cautions: Hypertension, Cancer
Myrtle M/BCd (Astringe, Clear heat/Lung, Drain damp/lower, Smooth liver qi, Wei qi) Myrtaceae
Cautions: Yang deficiency, Cold

BI SYNDROME

Top Warming..

Camphor THot (Bi/expel wind damp, Invigorate blood, Open orifice, Parasites, Resolve phlegm) Lauraceae
Cautions: Pregnancy, Epilepsy, Can irritate mucous membranes, Toxicity

Spruce T/MW (Bi/expel wind cold, Calm the shen, Stop coughing, Tonify qi, Tonify yang, Wei qi, Other: Helps kidneys graps lung qi) Pinaceae
Caution: May irritate the skin

Top Cooling...

Lemon TCd (Bi/damp Invigorate blood, Clear heat/liver/GB/stomach, Spleen qi, Wei qi, Other: Break up stones) Rutaceae
Cautions: Photosensitive

Sweet Marjoram T/MC (Bi/expel damp hot, Clear heat/liver, Food stasis, Regulate qi, Release exterior, Smooth liver qi, Stop coughing)
Lamiaceae/Labiatae
Cautions: Asthma, Pregnancy

Middle Warming...

Birch MW (Bi/expel wind damp cold, Clear Heat, Drain damp, Release exterior, Other: Open joints) Betulaceae
Cautions: Kidney toxicity, Kidney deficiency, May thin the blood, Pregnancy, Breastfeeding

Coriander MW (Bi/expel wind damp cold, Nourish yin/liver, Spleen qi, Tonify qi/kidney, Wei qi) Apiaceae/Umbelliferae
Cautions: Pregnancy, Can be photosensitive

Hyssop MW(Bi/expel damp cold, Invigorate blood, Spleen qi, Tonify qi/lung/heart, Tonify yang) Lamiaceae/Labiatae
Cautions: Neurotoxic, Liver wind, Glaucoma, Cancer, Pregnancy, Children, Excessive use can cause asthma, seizures, hypertension

Litsea MW (Bi/expel wind damp cold, Invigorate blood/lower, Regulate qi/lower, Release the exterior, Spleen qi, Tonify yang) Lauraceae
Cautions: Yin deficiency with heat

Oregano MW (Bi/expel wind damp cold, Move qi and blood, Open orifice, Parasites, Spleen qi, Wei qi, Other: Promotes menstruation)
Lamiaceae/Labiatae
Cautions: Heat/empty heat, Pregnancy, Liver toxicity

Spruce T/MW (Bi/expel wind cold, Calm the shen, Stop coughing, Tonify qi, Tonify yang, Wei qi, Other: Helps kidneys graps lung qi) Pinaceae
Caution: May irritate the skin

Terebinth MW (Bi/expel wind damp cold, Release Exterior, Subdue wind) Pinaceae
Cautions: Yin deficiency/liver/kidney, Blood deficiency, Epilepsy

Thuja MW (Bi/expel damp cold/lower) Cupressaceae
Cautions: Neurotoxic, Pregnancy
Wintergreen MW (Bi/expel wind damp hot, Release the exterior, Smooth liver qi) Ericaceae
Cautions: Kidney toxicity in overuse, Pregnancy
Middle Cooling..
Cajeput MC (Bi/Expel damp hot, Drain damp/lower jiao, Move qi and blood, Parasites, Release exterior, Tonify qi/lung) Myrtaceae
Celery Seed MC (Bi/wind damp, Clear fire toxin, Drain damp, Food stasis, Nourish yin/liver, Regulate qi, Smooth liver qi, Spleen qi, Tonify qi/kidney) Apiaceae/Umbelliferae
Cautions: Estrogenic, Photosensitive, Pregnancy, Breastfeeding
Fir MC (Bi/expel damp hot, Clear heat, Dry damp/lower, Resolve phlegm/damp, Stop coughing, Tonify qi/lung, Other: Help kidneys grasp qi) Pinaceae
Galbanum M/BC (Bi/expel damp hot, Calm the shen, Smooth liver qi, Tonify qi/lung) Apiaceae/Umbelliferae
Niaouli MC (Bi/wind damp/lower, Invigorate blood, Parasites, Release the exterior, Spleen qi, Tonify qi/lung/kidney, Wei qi) Myrtaceae
Cautions: Pregnancy, Children
Sweet Marjoram T/MC (Bi/expel damp hot, Clear heat/liver, Food stasis, Regulate qi, Release exterior, Smooth liver qi, Stop coughing) Lamiaceae/Labiatae
Cautions: Asthma, Pregnancy
Base Warming..
Benzoin BW (Bi/expel damp cold, Drain damp/lower, Spleen qi, Stop coughing, Tonify yang/spleen, Other: Diffuse lung qi) Styracaceae
Cautions: Heat, Empty heat
Cinnamon BHot (Astringe/blood, Bi/expel wind damp, Drain damp, Invigorate blood, Nourish blood, Parasites, Spleen qi, Tonify qi, Tonify yang, Warm interior to expel cold, Wei qi, Other: Regulate menstruation) Lauraceae
Cautions: Heat/empty heat, Mucous membranes, Pregnancy, May sensitize skin, Kidney, Liver toxicity, May prevent coagulation
Styrax BW (Bi/expel wind damp cold, Food stasis, Invigorate blood, Open Portals, Parasites, Resolve phlegm/turbid, Other: Promote menstruation) Styracaceae
Cautions: Pregnancy, Yang collapse, High fever
Base Cooling..
Galbanum M/BC (Bi/expel damp hot, Calm the shen, Smooth liver qi, Tonify qi/lung,) Apiaceae/Umbelliferae

Helichrysum BC (Bi/expel damp hot, Clear heat/Lung/Liver/Fire Toxin, Cool the blood, Move qi and blood, Nourish blood, Smooth liver qi, Wei qi) Asteracea/Compositae
Cautions: Yang deficiency

CALM THE SHEN

Top Warming..
Spruce T/MW (Bi/expel wind cold, Calm the shen, Stop coughing, Tonify qi, Tonify yang, Wei qi, Other: Helps kidneys grasp lung qi) Pinaceae
Caution: May irritate the skin
Top Neutral..
Geranium T/MN (Astringe/lower, Calm the shen, Cool the blood, Food stasis, Nourish yin, Parasites, Smooth liver qi, Spleen qi, Tonify qi/kidney, Other: Regulates menses) Gereniaceae
Cautions: Estrogenic, Pregnancy
Top Cooling..
Lavender T/MC (Calm the Shen, Clear heat/lung/liver, Nourish yin, Parasites, Regulate qi, Release the exterior, Smooth liver qi, Tonify qi/heart, Tonify yang/heart, Other: Diffuse lung qi) Lamiaceae/Labiatae
Mandarin TC (Calm the Shen, Food stasis, Regulate qi, Spleen qi, Subdue wind) Rutaceae
Petitgrain T/MC (Calm the shen, Drain damp, Regulate qi/chest, Smooth liver qi) Rutaceae
Spearmint T/MC (Calm the shen, Release the exterior, Smooth liver qi, Spleen qi, Wei qi, Other: Relieve itch) Lamiaceae/Labiatae
Cautions: Neurotoxic, Pregnancy, Mucous membranes
Middle Warming..
Spruce T/MW (Bi/expel wind cold, Calm the shen, Stop coughing, Tonify qi, Tonify yang, Wei qi, Other: Helps kidneys grasp lung qi) Pinaceae
Caution: May irritate the skin
Middle Neutral..
Geranium T/MN (Astringe/lower, Calm the shen, Cool the blood, Food stasis, Nourish yin, Parasites, Smooth liver qi, Spleen qi, Tonify qi/kidney, Other: Regulates menses) Gereniaceae
Cautions: Estrogenic, Pregnancy
Middle Cooling..
Galbanum M/BC (Bi/expel damp hot, Calm the shen, Smooth liver qi, Tonify qi/lung,) Apiaceae/Umbelliferae
German Chamomile MC (Calm the shen, Clear heat/liver/stomach/heart, Drain Damp, Nourish yin/heart, Smoothes Liver Qi, Spleen qi, Subdue wind, Tonify qi/Lung) Asteraceae/Compositae
Lavender T/MC (Calm the Shen, Clear heat/lung/liver, Nourish yin, Parasites, Regulate qi, Release the exterior, Smooth liver qi, Tonify qi/heart, Tonify yang/heart, Other: Diffuse lung qi) Lamiaceae/Labiatae

Mimosa MCold (Calm the shen, Clear heat/fire toxin, Cool the blood) Mimosaceae
Cautions: Cold or Deficient yang
Petitgrain T/MC (Calm the shen, Drain damp, Regulate qi/chest, Smooth liver qi) Rutaceae
Roman Chamomille MC (Calm the Shen, Clear heat/liver, Nourish blood, Nourish yin/liver, Regulate qi, Smooth liver qi, Subdue wind) Asteraceae/Compositae
Cautions: Yang deficiency, Ragweed allergy
Spearmint T/MC (Calm the shen, Release the exterior, Smooth liver qi, Spleen qi, Wei qi, Other: Relieve itch) Lamiaceae/Labiatae
Cautions: Neurotoxic, Pregnancy, Mucous membranes
Ylang Ylang M/BC (Calm the Shen, Clear heat/heart fire, Cool the blood, Nourish yin/heart/kidney, Tonifies qi/kidney, Wei qi) Annonaceae
Cautions: Yang deficiency, Cold
Base Warming...
Angelica BW (Calm the shen, Invigorate blood, Nourish blood, Smooth liver qi, Spleen qi, Tonify qi/lung, Wei qi, Other: Ease cough, Expel phlegm, Open the diaphragm) Apiaceae/Umbelliferae
Cautions: Photosensitive, Pregnancy, Diabetes
Balsam of Peru BW (Calm the Shen, Moves qi and blood, Parasites, Resolve phlegm, Tonifies Qi/Heart, Wei qi) Fabaceae
Cautions: May cause sensitization, Pregnancy, Breastfeeding
Vanilla BsW (Calm the Shen, Tonify qi/kidney, Other: Release suppressed emotion) Orchidaceae
Base Cooling...
Frankincense BsCd (Calm the shen, Clear heat/Lung/Stomach, Dry damp, Nourish blood/liver, Resolve phlegm, Strongly move qi and blood, Tonify qi/lung, Other: Reduce swelling) Berceraceae
Cautions: Pregnancy
Galbanum M/BC (Bi/expel damp hot, Calm the shen, Smooth liver qi, Tonify qi/lung,) Apiaceae/Umbelliferae
Narcissus BC (Calm the Shen, Other: Harmonize kidneys and heart) Amaryllidaceae
Cautions: Yang deficiency, Cold
Sandalwood BsC (Calm the Shen, Clear heat/Lower Jiao, Dry damp, Nourish yin, Moves qi and blood, Other: Opens diaphragm) Santalaceae
Spikenard BC (Calms the shen, Clear heat/Heart, Nourish yin/heart, Smooths liver qi, Subdue wind) Valerianaceae
Cautions: Exogenous conditions

Vetiver BC (Calm the Shen, Clear heat, Cool the blood, Invigorate blood, Nourish blood, Nourish yin, Smooth liver qi, Spleen qi, Tonify qi/heart) Gramineae

Violet BC (Calm the Shen, Clear heat/lung/fire toxin, Tonify qi/lung/heart, Other: Harmonize heart and kidney) Violaceae
Cautions: Yang deficiency, Cold

Ylang Ylang M/BC (Calm the Shen, Clear heat/heart fire, Cool the blood, Nourish yin/heart/kidney, Tonifies qi/kidney, Wei qi) Annonaceae
Cautions: Yang deficiency, Cold

CLEAR HEAT

Top Cooling...
Bergamot T/MsC (Clear heat/fire toxin, Drain damp, Food stagnation, Regulate qi, Release exterior, Smooth liver qi, Wei qi) Rutacae
Cautions: Photosensitive
Blue Yarrow TC (Clear Heat, Moves qi and blood, Tonifies qi/heart)
Cautions: Pregnancy
Lavender T/MC (Calm the Shen, Clear heat/lung/liver, Nourish yin, Parasites, Regulate qi, Release the exterior, Smooth liver qi, Tonify qi/heart, Tonify yang/heart, Other: Diffuse lung qi) Lamiaceae/Labiatae
Lemon TCd (Bi/damp, Invigorate blood, Clear heat/liver/GB/stomach, Spleen qi, Wei qi, Other: Break up stones) Rutaceae
Cautions: Photosensitive
Lemon Verbena TC (Clear heat/Heart/Liver, Smooth liver qi) Lamiaceae/Labiatae
Cautions: Mildly photosensitive
Orange TC (Clear heat/Heart, Food stasis, Regulate qi, Release exterior, Smooth liver qi, Spleen qi, Other: Clear heart fire) Rutaceae
Caution: Photosensitive
Palmarosa TC (Clear heat, Drain damp/lower, Nourish yin, Release the exterior, Smooth liver qi, Other: Clear damp heat skin outbreaks) Poaceae
Peppermint T/MC (Clear heat, Open portals, Regulate qi, Release exterior, Smooth liver qi, Spleen qi, Tonify qi/lung, Other: Move wei qi, Relieve itch) Lamiaceae/Labiatae
Cautions: Young children, Cardiac fibrillation, Epilepsy, Mucous membranes, Neurotoxic
Rosalina TC (Clear heat/stomach, Release the exterior) Myrtaceae
Caution: Pregnancy
Sage T/MC (Clear heat/stomach, Nourish yin, Release exterior, Resolve phlegm, Tonifies Qi/kidney, Other: Promote bile, Wei qi)
Lamiaceae/Labiatae
Cautions: May be estrogenic, Seizures, Pregnancy, Tisserand recommends avoiding Sage in aromatherapy.
Sweet Marjoram T/MC (Bi/expel damp hot, Clear heat/liver, Food stasis, Regulate qi, Release exterior, Smooth liver qi, Stop coughing)
Lamiaceae/Labiatae
Cautions: Asthma, Pregnancy

Middle Warming..

Birch MW (Bi/expel wind damp cold, Clear Heat, Drain damp, Release exterior, Other: Open joints) Betulaceae
Cautions: Kidney toxicity, Kidney deficiency, May thin the blood, Pregnancy, Breastfeeding

Middle Cooling...

Anise MC (Clear heat, Food stagnation, Regulate qi, Smooth liver qi, Stop cough, Other: Promote lactation) Apiaceae/Umbelliferae
Cautions: Mild estrogenic, Yin deficiency, Cancer, Pregnancy

Bergamot T/MsC (Clear heat/fire toxin, Drain damp, Food stagnation, Regulate qi, Release exterior, Smooth liver qi, Wei qi) Rutacae
Cautions: Photosensitive

Celery Seed MC (Bi/wind damp, Clear fire toxin, Drain damp, Food stasis, Nourish yin/liver, Regulate qi, Smooth liver qi, Spleen qi, Tonify qi/kidney) Apiaceae/Umbelliferae
Cautions: Estrogenic, Photosensitive, Pregnancy, Breastfeeding

Clary Sage MC (Clear heat/stomach, Cool the blood, Nourish yin, Smooth liver qi, Spleen qi, Subdue wind, Tonify qi/heart/lung, Other: Clear empty heat, Encourages labor, Regulates menses, Running piglet qi) Lamiaceae/Labiatae
Cautions: Estrogenic, Can be narcotic in larger doses, Cancer, Pregancy, Alcohol consumption

Cypress M/BsC (Astringe, Clear heat/lung, Move qi and blood, Stop coughing, Other: Ascend spleen qi, Assist kidney to grasp lung qi) Cupressaceae
Cautions: Hypertension, Cancer

Fir MC (Bi/expel damp hot, Clear heat, Dry damp/lower, Resolve phlegm/damp, Stop coughing, Tonify qi/lung, Other: Help kidneys grasp qi) Pinaceae

German Chamomile MC (Calm the shen, Clear heat/liver/stomach/heart, Drain Damp, Nourish yin/heart, Smoothes Liver Qi, Spleen qi, Subdue wind, Tonify qi/Lung) Asteraceae/Compositae

Hyssop Linalool MC (Clear heat/lung) Lamiaceae/Labiatae
Cautions: Yang deficiency, Ragweed allergy

Lavender T/MC (Calm the Shen, Clear heat/lung/liver, Nourish yin, Parasites, Regulate qi, Release the exterior, Smooth liver qi, Tonify qi/heart, Tonify yang/heart, Other: Diffuse lung qi) Lamiaceae/Labiatae

Lavendin MC (Clear heat/lung/liver, Smooth liver qi)Lamiaceae/Labiatae
Cautions: Yang deficiency, (Not toxic when diluted.)

Melissa MC (Astringe/blood, Clear heat/liver/heart/wei, Cools the blood, Food stasis, Parasites, Regulate qi, Release the exterior, Smooth liver qi, Other: Open and relax the chest) Lamiaceae/Labiatae
Cautions: Can be sensitizing in high doses.

Mimosa MCold (Calm the shen, Clear heat/fire toxin, Cool the blood) Mimosaceae
Cautions: Cold or Deficient yang
Myrtle M/BCd (Astringe, Clear heat/Lung, Drain damp/lower, Smooth liver qi, Wei qi) Myrtaceae
Cautions: Yang deficiency, Cold
Neroli M/BC (Clear heat/Heart/fire toxin, Spleen qi, Tonify qi) Rutaceae
Peppermint T/MC (Clear heat, Open portals, Regulate qi, Release exterior, Smooth liver qi, Spleen qi, Tonify qi/lung, Other: Move wei qi, Relieve itch) Lamiaceae/Labiatae
Cautions: Young children, Cardiac fibrillation, Epilepsy, Mucous membranes, Neurotoxic
Ravensare MC (Clear heat/lung, Release exterior) Lauraceae
Roman Chamomille MC (Calm the Shen, Clear heat/liver, Nourish blood, Nourish yin/liver, Regulate qi, Smooth liver qi, Subdue wind) Asteraceae/Compositae
Cautions: Yang deficiency, Ragweed allergy
Sage T/MC (Clear heat/stomach, Nourish yin, Release exterior, Resolve phlegm, Tonifies Qi/kidney, Other: Promote bile, Wei qi) Lamiaceae/Labiatae
Cautions: May be estrogenic, Seizures, Pregnancy, Tisserand recommends avoiding Sage in aromatherapy.
Sweet Marjoram T/MC (Bi/expel damp hot, Clear heat/liver, Food stasis, Regulate qi, Release exterior, Smooth liver qi, Stop coughing) Lamiaceae/Labiatae
Cautions: Asthma, Pregnancy
Tea Tree MC (Clear heat, Dry damp, Invigorate blood, Parasites, Release exterior, Tonify qi, Wei qi) Myraceae
Thyme Linalool MC (Clear heat/lung/stomach, Parasites, Tonify qi) Lamiaceae/Labiatae
Cautions: Glaucoma
Yarrow MCold (Clear heat, Moves qi and blood, Smoothes liver qi, Spleen qi, Tonifies qi/heart/kidney, Other: Ascend spleen qi, Promote sweating) Asteracea/Compositae
Cautions: Neurotoxic, Children, Pregnancy, Ragweed allergy
Ylang Ylang M/BC (Calm the Shen, Clear heat/heart fire, Cool the blood, Nourish yin/heart/kidney, Tonifies qi/kidney, Wei qi) Annonaceae
Cautions: Yang deficiency, Cold
Base Warming..
Patchouli BsW (Clear summer heat, Release the exterior, Strongly tonify spleen qi, Other: Release suppressed emotion) Lamiaceae/Labiatae

---

Base Neutral..

Rose BN (Clear heat/liver, Cool the blood, Invigorate blood, Nourish yin, Open orifice, Smooth liver qi, Other: Harmonize kidney/heart, Promote bile) Roseaceae

Base Cooling..

Cedarwood BC (Clear heat/Lung, Dry damp/lower, Spleen qi, Tonify qi/lung, Tonify yang/kidney/spleen, Other: Relieve itch) Cupressaceae
Cautions: Pregnancy, Prepubescent children

Cypress M/BsC (Astringe, Clear heat/lung, Move qi and blood, Stop coughing, Other: Ascend spleen qi, Assist kidney to grasp lung qi) Cupressaceae
Cautions: Hypertension, Cancer

Frankincense BsCd (Calm the shen, Clear heat/Lung/Stomach, Dry damp, Nourish blood/liver, Resolve phlegm, Strongly move qi and blood, Tonify qi/lung, Other: Reduce swelling) Berceraceae
Cautions: Pregnancy

Helichrysum BC (Bi/expel damp hot, Clear heat/Lung/Liver/Fire Toxin, Cool the blood, Move qi and blood, Nourish blood, Smooth liver qi, Wei qi) Asteracea/Compositae
Cautions: Yang deficiency

Inula BsC (Clear heat/Lung, Drain/transform damp/upper, Stop coughing, Tonify qi/heart, Wei qi) Asteracea/Compositae
Cautions: Toxicity

Jasmine BC (Clear heat/Liver, Nourish yin, Other: Clear empty heat, Promote childbirth) Oleaceae
Cautions: Yang deficiency

Lovage BCold (Clear heat/stomach/kidney, Drain damp, Resolve phlegm, Spleen qi) Apiaceae/Umbelliferae
Cautions: Photosensitive, Toxic

Marigold BC (Clear heat, Resolve hot phlegm, Other: Promote bile secretion) Asteracea/Compositae
Cautions: Photosensitive, Toxic, Epilepsy, Pregnancy

Myrrh BC (Clear heat/Lung/Stomach, Dry damp, Move qi and blood, Spleen qi, Other: Promotes healing of wounds) Burseraceae
Cautions: Pregnancy, Uterine bleeding

Myrtle M/BCd (Astringe, Clear heat/Lung, Drain damp/lower, Smooth liver qi, Wei qi) Myrtaceae
Cautions: Yang deficiency, Cold

Neroli M/BC (Clear heat/Heart/fire toxin, Spleen qi, Tonify qi) Rutaceae

Sandalwood BsC (Calm the Shen, Clear heat/Lower Jiao, Dry damp, Nourish yin, Moves qi and blood, Other: Opens diaphragm) Santalaceae

Spikenard BC (Calms the shen, Clear heat/Heart, Nourish yin/heart, Smooths liver qi, Subdue wind) Valerianaceae
Cautions: Exogenous conditions
Vetiver BC (Calm the Shen, Clear heat, Cool the blood, Invigorate blood, Nourish blood, Nourish yin, Smooth liver qi, Spleen qi, Tonify qi/heart) Gramineae
Violet BC (Calm the Shen, Clear heat/lung/fire toxin, Tonify qi/lung/heart, Other: Harmonize heart and kidney) Violaceae
Cautions: Yang deficiency, Cold
Ylang Ylang M/BC (Calm the Shen, Clear heat/heart fire, Cool the blood, Nourish yin/heart/kidney, Tonifies qi/kidney, Wei qi) Annonaceae
Cautions: Yang deficiency, Cold

COOL THE BLOOD

Top Neutral...

Geranium T/MN (Astringe/lower, Calm the shen, Cool the blood, Food stasis, Nourish yin, Parasites, Smooth liver qi, Spleen qi, Tonify qi/kidney, Other: Regulates menses) Gereniaceae
Cautions: Estrogenic, Pregnancy

Middle Neutral...

Geranium T/MN (Astringe/lower, Calm the shen, Cool the blood, Food stasis, Nourish yin, Parasites, Smooth liver qi, Spleen qi, Tonify qi/kidney, Other: Regulates menses) Gereniaceae
Cautions: Estrogenic, Pregnancy

Middle Cooling..

Clary Sage MC (Clear heat/stomach, Cool the blood, Nourish yin, Smooth liver qi, Spleen qi, Subdue wind, Tonify qi/heart/lung, Other: Clear empty heat, Encourages labor, Regulates menses, Running piglet qi) Lamiaceae/Labiatae
Cautions: Estrogenic, Can be narcotic in larger doses, Cancer, Pregnancy, Alcohol consumption

Melissa MC (Astringe/blood, Clear heat/liver/heart/wei, Cools the blood, Food stasis, Parasites, Regulate qi, Release the exterior, Smooth liver qi, Other: Open and relax the chest) Lamiaceae/Labiatae
Cautions: Can be sensitizing in high doses.

Mimosa MCold (Calm the shen, Clear heat/fire toxin, Cool the blood) Mimosaceae
Cautions: Cold or Deficient yang

Ylang Ylang M/BC (Calm the Shen, Clear heat/heart fire, Cool the blood, Nourish yin/heart/kidney, Tonifies qi/kidney, Wei qi) Annonaceae
Cautions: Yang deficiency, Cold

Base Neutral...

Rose BN (Clear heat/liver, Cool the blood, Invigorate blood, Nourish yin, Open orifice, Smooth liver qi, Other: Harmonize kidney/heart, Promote bile) Roseaceae

Base Cooling...

Helichrysum BC (Bi/expel damp hot, Clear heat/Lung/Liver/Fire Toxin, Cool the blood, Move qi and blood, Nourish blood, Smooth liver qi, Wei qi) Asteracea/Compositae
Cautions: Yang deficiency

Vetiver BC (Calm the Shen, Clear heat, Cool the blood, Invigorate blood, Nourish blood, Nourish yin, Smooth liver qi, Spleen qi, Tonify qi/heart) Gramineae

Ylang Ylang M/BC (Calm the Shen, Clear heat/heart fire, Cool the blood, Nourish yin/heart/kidney, Tonifies qi/kidney, Wei qi) Annonaceae
Cautions: Yang deficiency, Cold

DRAIN DAMP

Top Warming...

Eucalyptus Globulus T/MW (Drain damp, Move qi and blood, Parasites, Release the exterior, Wei qi) Myrtaceae
Cautions: Children and babies

Eucalyptus Radiata TW (Drain damp, Resolve Phlegm, Tonify qi, Wei qi) Myrtaceae

Grapefruit TsWd (Drain damp, Food stasis, Regulate qi, Resolve phlegm, Smooth liver qi, Other, Promote bile production) Rutaceae
Cautions: Photosensitive, Heat patterns

Top Cooling...

Bergamot T/MsC (Clear heat/fire toxin, Drain damp, Food stagnation, Regulate qi, Release exterior, Smooth liver qi, Wei qi) Rutacae
Cautions: Photosensitive

Eucalyptus Citriodora TC (Drain damp, Move qi and blood, Wei qi,) Myrtaceae
Cautions: Children

Eucalyptus Smithii TC (Drain damp, Resolve Phlegm, Tonifies Qi, Wei qi) Myrtaceae
Cautions: Children 3 and under, Pregnancy

Palmarosa TC (Clear heat, Drain damp/lower, Nourish yin, Release the exterior, Smooth liver qi, Other: Clear damp heat skin outbreaks) Poaceae

Petitgrain T/MC (Calm the shen, Drain damp, Regulate qi/chest, Smooth liver qi) Rutaceae

Middle Warming...

Birch MW (Bi/expel wind damp cold, Clear Heat, Drain damp, Release exterior, Other: Open joints) Betulaceae
Cautions: Kidney toxicity, Kidney deficiency, May thin the blood, Pregnancy, Breastfeeding

Eucalyptus Globulus T/MW (Drain damp, Move qi and blood, Parasites, Release the exterior, Wei qi) Myrtaceae
Cautions: Children and babies

Fennel MW (Drain damp, Nourish yin, Spleen qi, Tonify qi/lung, Tonify yang) Apiaceae/Umbelliferae Cautions: Estrogenic, Heat, Interior wind, Pregnancy, Cancer, Hypothyroidism

Juniper MW (Drain damp, Invigorate blood, Resolve phlegm, Spleen qi, Tonify yang/strongly, Other: Promote menstruation) Cupressaceae
Cautions: Kidney yin deficiency, Kidney toxicity, Pregnancy

Parsley MW (Drain damp/lower, Invigorate blood, Regulate qi/stomach, Other: Abortion, Childbirth, Promote menstruation) Umbelliferae
Cautions: Neurotoxic, Liver toxic, Pregnancy, Breastfeeding

Middle Cooling..

Bergamot T/MsC (Clear heat/fire toxin, Drain damp, Food stagnation, Regulate qi, Release exterior, Smooth liver qi, Wei qi) Rutacae
Cautions: Photosensitive

Cajeput MC (Bi/Expel damp hot, Drain damp/lower jiao, Move qi and blood, Parasites, Release exterior, Tonify qi/lung) Myrtaceae

Carrot (seed) MC (Drain damp, Nourish blood, Nourish yin/liver, Smooth liver qi) Apiaceae/Umbelliferae

Celery Seed MC (Bi/wind damp, Clear fire toxin, Drain damp, Food stasis, Nourish yin/liver, Regulate qi, Smooth liver qi, Spleen qi, Tonify qi/kidney) Apiaceae/Umbelliferae
Cautions: Estrogenic, Photosensitive, Pregnancy, Breastfeeding

Fir MC (Bi/expel damp hot, Clear heat, Dry damp/lower, Resolve phlegm/damp, Stop coughing, Tonify qi/lung, Other: Help kidneys grasp qi) Pinaceae Petitgrain TMC (Calm the shen, Drain damp, Regulate qi/chest, Smooth liver qi) Rutacae

German Chamomile MC (Calm the shen, Clear heat/liver/stomach/heart, Drain Damp, Nourish yin/heart, Smoothes Liver Qi, Spleen qi, Subdue wind, Tonify qi/Lung) Asteraceae/Compositae

Tea Tree MC (Clear heat, Dry damp, Invigorate blood, Parasites, Release exterior, Tonify qi, Wei qi) Myraceae

Base Warming...

Benzoin BW (Bi/expel damp cold, Drain damp/lower, Spleen qi, Stop coughing, Tonify yang/spleen, Other: Diffuse lung qi) Styracaceae
Cautions: Heat, Empty heat

Cinnamon BHot (Astringe/blood, Bi/expel wind damp, Drain damp, Invigorate blood, Nourish blood, Parasites, Spleen qi, Tonify qi, Tonify yang, Warm interior to expel cold, Wei qi, Other: Regulate menstruation) Lauraceae
Cautions: Heat/empty heat, Mucous membranes, Pregnancy, May sensitize skin, Kidney, Liver toxicity, May prevent coagulation

Dill BW (Drain damp, Food stasis, Invigorate blood, Spleen qi, Stop coughing, Other: Lactation, Promote bile secretion) Apiaceae/Umbelliferae
Cautions: Heat/empty heat, Yin deficiency, Liver wind/ascending yang, Pregnancy

Base Cooling...

Cedarwood BC (Clear heat/Lung, Dry damp/lower, Spleen qi, Tonify qi/lung, Tonify yang/kidney/spleen, Other: Relieve itch) Cupressaceae
Cautions: Pregnancy, Prepubescent children

Frankincense BsCd (Calm the shen, Clear heat/Lung/Stomach, Dry damp, Nourish blood/liver, Resolve phlegm, Strongly move qi and blood, Tonify qi/lung, Other: Reduce swelling) Berceraceae
Cautions: Pregnancy

Inula BsC (Clear heat/Lung, Drain/transform damp/upper, Stop coughing, Tonify qi/heart, Wei qi) Asteracea/Compositae
Cautions: Toxicity
Lovage BCold (Clear heat/stomach/kidney, Drain damp, Resolve phlegm, Spleen qi) Apiaceae/Umbelliferae
Cautions: Photosensitive, Toxic
Myrrh BC (Clear heat/Lung/Stomach, Dry damp, Move qi and blood, Spleen qi, Other: Promotes healing of wounds) Burseraceae
Cautions: Pregnancy, Uterine bleeding
Sandalwood BsC (Calm the Shen, Clear heat/Lower Jiao, Dry damp, Nourish yin, Moves qi and blood, Other: Opens diaphragm) Santalaceae

FOOD STAGNATION

Top Warming...

Basil T/MW (Food stasis, Nourish yin/liver, Release the exterior, Spleen qi, Tonify qi//kidney, Tonify yang, Wei qi, Other: Promote lactation, Relieve uterine contraction) Lamiaceae/Labiatae
Cautions: Use in small doses, Pregnancy

Grapefruit TsWd (Drain damp, Food stasis, Regulate qi, Resolve phlegm, Smooth liver qi, Other, Promote bile production) Rutaceae
Cautions: Photosensitive, Heat patterns

Pennyroyal T/MW (Food stasis, Spleen qi, Stop coughing, Other: Promote bile, Regulate menses) Lamiaceae/Labiatae
Cautions: Pregnancy

Top Neutral..

Geranium T/MN (Astringe/lower, Calm the shen, Cool the blood, Food stasis, Nourish yin, Parasites, Smooth liver qi, Spleen qi, Tonify qi/kidney, Other: Regulates menses) Gereniaceae
Cautions: Estrogenic, Pregnancy

Top Cooling...

Bay Laurel TsC (Food stasis, Regulate qi/stomach, Resolve hot phlegm) Lauraceae
Cautions: Narcotic in large doses, Pregnancy

Bergamot T/MsC (Clear heat/fire toxin, Drain damp, Food stagnation, Regulate qi, Release exterior, Smooth liver qi, Wei qi) Rutacae
Cautions: Photosensitive

Bitter Orange TCold (Food stagnation, Regulate qi/liver/stomach, Smooth liver qi, Spleen qi) Rutacae Cautions: Photosensitive, Qi deficiency, Cold stomach

Mandarin TC (Calm the Shen, Food stasis, Regulate qi, Spleen qi, Subdue wind) Rutaceae

Orange TC (Clear heat/Heart, Food stasis, Regulate qi, Release exterior, Smooth liver qi, Spleen qi, Other: Clear heart fire) Rutaceae
Caution: Photosensitive

Sweet Marjoram T/MC (Bi/expel damp hot, Clear heat/liver, Food stasis, Regulate qi, Release exterior, Smooth liver qi, Stop coughing) Lamiaceae/Labiatae
Cautions: Asthma, Pregnancy

Middle Warming...

Basil T/MW (Food stasis, Nourish yin/liver, Release the exterior, Spleen qi, Tonify qi//kidney, Tonify yang, Wei qi, Other: Promote lactation, Relieve uterine contraction) Lamiaceae/Labiatae
Cautions: Use in small doses, Pregnancy

Cardamom MW (Food stasis, Invigorate blood, Regulate qi, Spleen qi, Stop coughing, Tonify qi/Lung) Zingiberaceae
Cautions: Yin deficiency, Blood deficiency
Pennyroyal T/MW (Food stasis, Spleen qi, Stop coughing, Other: Promote bile, Regulate menses) Lamiaceae/Labiatae
Cautions: Pregnancy
Tarragon MW (Food stasis, Moves qi and blood, Nourish Blood, Parasites, Spleen qi, Tonify Qi/heart, Other: Promote menstruation) Asteraceae
Cautions: Pregnancy, Cancer
Middle Neutral..
Geranium T/MN (Astringe/lower, Calm the shen, Cool the blood, Food stasis, Nourish yin, Parasites, Smooth liver qi, Spleen qi, Tonify qi/kidney, Other: Regulates menses) Gereniaceae
Cautions: Estrogenic, Pregnancy
Middle Cooling..
Anise MC (Clear heat, Food stagnation, Regulate qi, Smooth liver qi, Stop cough, Other: Promote lactation) Apiaceae/Umbelliferae
Cautions: Mild estrogenic, Yin deficiency, Cancer, Pregnancy
Bergamot T/MsC (Clear heat/fire toxin, Drain damp, Food stagnation, Regulate qi, Release exterior, Smooth liver qi, Wei qi) Rutacae
Cautions: Photosensitive
Celery Seed MC (Bi/wind damp, Clear fire toxin, Drain damp, Food stasis, Nourish yin/liver, Regulate qi, Smooth liver qi, Spleen qi, Tonify qi/kidney) Apiaceae/Umbelliferae
Cautions: Estrogenic, Photosensitive, Pregnancy, Breastfeeding
Melissa MC (Astringe/blood, Clear heat/liver/heart/wei, Cools the blood, Food stasis, Parasites, Regulate qi, Release the exterior, Smooth liver qi, Other: Open and relax the chest) Lamiaceae/Labiatae
Cautions: Can be sensitizing in high doses.
Sweet Marjoram T/MC (Bi/expel damp hot, Clear heat/liver, Food stasis, Regulate qi, Release exterior, Smooth liver qi, Stop coughing) Lamiaceae/Labiatae
Cautions: Asthma, Pregnancy
Base Warming...
Dill BW (Drain damp, Food stasis, Invigorate blood, Spleen qi, Stop coughing, Other: Lactation, Promote bile secretion) Apiaceae/Umbelliferae
Cautions: Heat/empty heat, Yin deficiency, Liver wind/ascending yang, Pregnancy
Styrax BW (Bi/expel wind damp cold, Food stasis, Invigorate blood, Open portals, Parasites, Resolve phlegm/turbid, Other: Promote menstruation) Styracaceae
Cautions: Pregnancy, Yang collapse, High fever

INVIGORATE BLOOD

Top Warming...
Camphor THot (Bi/expel wind damp, Invigorate blood, Open orifice, Parasites, Resolve phlegm) Lauraceae
Cautions: Pregnancy, Epilepsy, Can irritate mucous membranes, Toxicity
Eucalyptus Globulus T/MW (Drain damp, Move qi and blood, Parasites, Release the exterior, Wei qi) Myrtaceae
Cautions: Children and babies
Top Cooling...
Blue Yarrow TC (Clear Heat, Moves qi and blood, Tonifies qi/heart)
Cautions: Pregnancy
Eucalyptus Citriodora TC (Drain damp, Move qi and blood, Wei qi,) Myrtaceae
Cautions: Children
Tangerine TC (Nourish blood, Move qi and blood, Spleen qi) Rutaceae
Cautions: May be photosensitive
Middle Warming...
Cardamom MW (Food stasis, Invigorate blood, Regulate qi, Spleen qi, Stop coughing, Tonify qi/Lung) Zingiberaceae
Cautions: Yin deficiency, Blood deficiency
Cinnamon Leaf MW (Invigorate blood, Release exterior, Spleen qi, Other: Promote sweating, Stimulate childbirth) Lauraceae
Cautions: Heat/empty heat
Cumin MsW (Invigorate blood, Smooth liver qi, Spleen qi, Tonify qi/heart) Apiaceae/Umbelliferae
Cautions: Photosensitive, Pregnancy
Eucalyptus Globulus T/MW (Drain damp, Move qi and blood, Parasites, Release the exterior, Wei qi) Myrtaceae
Cautions: Children and babies
Ginger M/BHot (Invigorate blood, Parasites, Release exterior, Spleen qi, Tonify qi/lung/heart/kidney, Tonify yang, Warm interior to expel cold, Wei qi, Other: Harmonize blends) Zingiberaceae
Cautions: Heat/empty heat, Stomach fire
Hyssop MW(Bi/expel damp cold, Invigorate blood, Spleen qi, Tonify qi/lung/heart, Tonify yang) Lamiaceae/Labiatae
Cautions: Neurotoxic, Liver wind, Glaucoma, Cancer, Pregnancy, Children, Excessive use can cause asthma, Seizures, Hypertension
Juniper MW (Drain damp, Invigorate blood, Resolve phlegm, Spleen qi, Tonify yang/strongly, Other: Promote menstruation) Cupressaceae
Cautions: Kidney yin deficiency, Kidney toxicity, Pregnancy

Litsea MW (Bi/expel wind damp cold, Invigorate blood/lower, Regulate qi/lower, Release the exterior, Spleen qi, Tonify yang) Lauraceae
Cautions: Yin deficiency with heat

Nutmeg MW (Nourish blood, Move qi and blood, Spleen qi, Tonify yang/spleen/kidney, Warm interior to expel cold) Myristicaceae
Cautions: Diarrhea due to heat, Liver wind/ascending yang, Epilepsy, Liver toxicity, Pregnancy, High doses can produce delirium convulsions, Hallucinations, Dizziness, Fainting, Cancer

Onion MW (Invigorate blood, Parasites, Resolve phlegm, Warm interior to expel cold) Liliaceae
Cautions: Heat/empty heat

Oregano MW (Bi/expel wind damp cold, Move qi and blood, Open orifice, Parasites, Spleen qi, Wei qi, Other: Promotes menstruation) Lamiaceae/Labiatae
Cautions: Heat/empty heat, Pregnancy, Liver toxicity

Parsley MW (Drain damp/lower, Invigorate blood, Regulate qi/stomach, Other: Abortion, Childbirth, Promote menstruation) Umbelliferae
Cautions: Neurotoxic, Liver toxic, Pregnancy, Breastfeeding

Tarragon MW (Food stasis, Moves qi and blood, Nourish Blood, Parasites, Spleen qi, Tonify Qi/heart, Other: Promote menstruation) Asteraceae
Cautions: Pregnancy, Cancer

Middle Cooling...

Cajeput MC (Bi/Expel damp hot, Drain damp/lower jiao, Move qi and blood, Parasites, Release exterior, Tonify qi/lung) Myrtaceae

Cypress M/BsC (Astringe, Clear heat/lung, Move qi and blood, Stop coughing, Other: Ascend spleen qi, Assist kidney to grasp lung qi) Cupressaceae
Cautions: Hypertension, Cancer

Niaouli MC (Bi/wind damp/lower, Invigorate blood, Parasites, Release the exterior, Spleen qi, Tonify qi/lung/kidney, Wei qi) Myrtaceae
Cautions: Pregnancy, Children

Tea Tree MC (Clear heat, Dry damp, Invigorate blood, Parasites, Release exterior, Tonify qi, Wei qi) Myraceae

Yarrow MCold (Clear heat, Moves qi and blood, Smoothes liver qi, Spleen qi, Tonifies qi/heart/kidney, Other: Ascend spleen qi, Promote sweating) Asteracea/Compositae
Cautions: Neurotoxic, Children, Pregnancy, Ragweed allergy

Base Warming...

Angelica BW (Calm the shen, Invigorate blood, Nourish blood, Smooth liver qi, Spleen qi, Tonify qi/lung, Wei qi, Other: Ease cough, Expel phlegm, Open the diaphragm) Apiaceae/Umbelliferae
Cautions: Photosensitive, Pregnancy, Diabetes

Balsam of Peru BW (Calm the Shen, Moves qi and blood, Parasites, Resolve phlegm, Tonifies Qi/Heart, Wei qi) Fabaceae
Cautions: May cause sensitization, Pregnancy, Breastfeeding
Cinnamon BHot (Astringe/blood, Bi/expel wind damp, Drain damp, Invigorate blood, Nourish blood, Parasites, Spleen qi, Tonify qi, Tonify yang, Warm interior to expel cold, Wei qi, Other: Regulate menstruation) Lauraceae
Cautions: Heat/empty heat, Mucous membranes, Pregnancy, May sensitize skin, Kidney, Liver toxicity, May prevent coagulation
Dill BW (Drain damp, Food stasis, Invigorate blood, Spleen qi, Stop coughing, Other: Lactation, Promote bile secretion) Apiaceae/Umbelliferae
Cautions: Heat/empty heat, Yin deficiency, Liver wind/ascending yang, Pregnancy
Elemi BWd (Invigorate blood/chest, Regulate qi/chest, Resolve phlegm) Berseraceae
Cautions: Pregnancy
Ginger M/BHot (Invigorate blood, Parasites, Release exterior, Spleen qi, Tonify qi/lung/heart/kidney, Tonify yang, Warm interior to expel cold, Wei qi, Other: Harmonize blends) Zingiberaceae
Cautions: Heat/empty heat, Stomach fire
Styrax BW (Bi/expel wind damp cold, Food stasis, Invigorate blood, Open portals, Parasites, Resolve phlegm/turbid, Other: Promote menstruation) Styracaceae
Cautions: Pregnancy, Yang collapse, High fever
Base Neutral..
Rose BN (Clear heat/liver, Cool the blood, Invigorate blood, Nourish yin, Open orifice, Smooth liver qi, Other: Harmonize kidney/heart, Promote bile) Roseaceae
Base Cooling...
Cypress M/BsC (Astringe, Clear heat/lung, Move qi and blood, Stop coughing, Other: Ascend spleen qi, Assist kidney to grasp lung qi) Cupressaceae
Cautions: Hypertension, Cancer
Frankincense BsCd (Calm the shen, Clear heat/Lung/Stomach, Dry damp, Nourish blood/liver, Resolve phlegm, Strongly move qi and blood, Tonify qi/lung, Other: Reduce swelling) Berceraceae
Cautions: Pregnancy
Helichrysum BC (Bi/expel damp hot, Clear heat/Lung/Liver/Fire Toxin, Cool the blood, Move qi and blood, Nourish blood, Smooth liver qi, Wei qi) Asteracea/Compositae
Cautions: Yang deficiency

Myrrh BC (Clear heat/Lung/Stomach, Dry damp, Move qi and blood, Spleen qi, Other: Promotes healing of wounds) Burseraceae
Cautions: Pregnancy, Uterine bleeding
Sandalwood BsC (Calm the Shen, Clear heat/Lower Jiao, Dry damp, Nourish yin, Moves qi and blood, Other: Opens diaphragm) Santalaceae
Vetiver BC (Calm the Shen, Clear heat, Cool the blood, Invigorate blood, Nourish blood, Nourish yin, Smooth liver qi, Spleen qi, Tonify qi/heart) Gramineae

NOURISH BLOOD

Top Warming...
Lemongrass TW (Nourish blood, Spleen qi, Tonify yang, Warm interior to expel cold, Wei qi) Graminae
Cautions: Heat/empty heat, Glaucoma, Children, Prostatic hyperplasia, Slight risk of sensitization
Rosemary T/MW (Nourish blood, Regulate qi, Release the exterior, Spleen qi, Tonify qi/kidney/heart, Tonify yang, Warm the interior to expel cold) Lamiaceae/Labiatae
Cautions: Heat/empty heat, Pregnancy, Children, Rebellious qi, Hypertension
Top Cooling..
Tangerine TC (Nourish blood, Move qi and blood, Spleen qi) Rutaceae
Cautions: May be photosensitive
Middle Warming..
Nutmeg MW (Nourish blood, Move qi and blood, Spleen qi, Tonify yang/spleen/kidney, Warm interior to expel cold) Myristicaceae
Cautions: Diarrhea due to heat, Liver wind/ascending yang, Epilepsy, Liver toxicity, Pregnancy, High doses can produce delirium convulsions, Hallucinations, Dizziness, Fainting, Cancer
Rosemary T/MW (Nourish blood, Regulate qi, Release the exterior, Spleen qi, Tonify qi/kidney/heart, Tonify yang, Warm the interior to expel cold) Lamiaceae/Labiatae
Cautions: Heat/empty heat, Pregnancy, Children, Rebellious qi, Hypertension
Savory MW (Nourish blood, Parasites, Resolve phlegm, Spleen qi, Tonify qi) Lamiaceae/Labiatae
Cautions: Heat/empty heat, Pregnancy
Tarragon MW (Food stasis, Moves qi and blood, Nourish Blood, Parasites, Spleen qi, Tonify Qi/heart, Other: Promote menstruation) Asteraceae
Cautions: Pregnancy, Cancer
Middle Cooling..
Carrot (seed) MC (Drain damp, Nourish blood, Nourish yin/liver, Smooth liver qi) Apiaceae/Umbelliferae
Roman Chamomille MC (Calm the Shen, Clear heat/liver, Nourish blood, Nourish yin/liver, Regulate qi, Smooth liver qi, Subdue wind) Asteraceae/Compositae
Cautions: Yang deficiency, Ragweed allergy
Thyme Geraniol MC (Nourish blood)
Cautions: Hypertension, May irritate skin, Mucous membranes

Base Warming..

Angelica BW (Calm the shen, Invigorate blood, Nourish blood, Smooth liver qi, Spleen qi, Tonifyqi/lung, Wei qi, Other: Ease cough, Expel phlegm, Open the diaphragm) Apiaceae/Umbelliferae

Cautions: Photosensitive, Pregnancy, Diabetes

Cinnamon BHot (Astringe/blood, Bi/expel wind damp, Drain damp, Invigorate blood, Nourish blood, Parasites, Spleen qi, Tonify qi, Tonify yang, Warm interior to expel cold, Wei qi, Other: Regulate menstruation) Lauraceae

Cautions: Heat/empty heat, Mucous membranes, Pregnancy, May sensitize skin, Kidney, Liver toxicity, May prevent coagulation

Valerian Root BW (Nourish blood, Nourish yin, Parasites, Regulate Qi, Subdue wind, Tonifies Qi/heart, Tonify Yang/heart, Wei qi) Valerianaceae

Cautions: Qi deficiency, Yang deficiency, Pregnancy, Children

Base Cooling..

Frankincense BsCd (Calm the shen, Clear heat/Lung/Stomach, Dry damp, Nourish blood/liver, Resolve phlegm, Strongly move qi and blood, Tonify qi/lung, Other: Reduce swelling) Berceraceae

Cautions: Pregnancy

Helichrysum BC (Bi/expel damp hot, Clear heat/Lung/Liver/Fire Toxin, Cool the blood, Move qi and blood, Nourish blood, Smooth liver qi, Wei qi) Asteracea/Compositae

Cautions: Yang deficiency

Vetiver BC (Calm the Shen, Clear heat, Cool the blood, Invigorate blood, Nourish blood, Nourish yin, Smooth liver qi, Spleen qi, Tonify qi/heart) Gramineae

NOURISH YIN

Top Warming..
Basil T/MW (Food stasis, Nourish yin/liver, Release the exterior, Spleen qi, Tonify qi//kidney, Tonify yang, Wei qi, Other: Promote lactation, Relieve uterine contraction) Lamiaceae/Labiatae
Cautions: Use in small doses, Pregnancy
Top Neutral..
Geranium T/MN (Astringe/lower, Calm the shen, Cool the blood, Food stasis, Nourish yin, Parasites, Smooth liver qi, Spleen qi, Tonify qi/kidney, Other: Regulates menses) Gereniaceae
Cautions: Estrogenic, Pregnancy
Top Cooling..
Lavender T/MC (Calm the Shen, Clear heat/lung/liver, Nourish yin, Parasites, Regulate qi, Release the exterior, Smooth liver qi, Tonify qi/heart, Tonify yang/heart, Other: Diffuse lung qi) Lamiaceae/Labiatae
Palmarosa TC (Clear heat, Drain damp/lower, Nourish yin, Release the exterior, Smooth liver qi, Other: Clear damp heat skin outbreaks) Poaceae
Sage T/MC (Clear heat/stomach, Nourish yin, Release exterior, Resolve phlegm, Tonifies qi/kidney, Other: Promote bile, Wei qi) Lamiaceae/Labiatae
Cautions: May be estrogenic, Seizures, Pregnancy, Tisserand recommends avoiding Sage in aromatherapy.
Middle Warming..
Basil T/MW (Food stasis, Nourish yin/liver, Release the exterior, Spleen qi, Tonify qi//kidney, Tonify yang, Wei qi, Other: Promote lactation, Relieve uterine contraction) Lamiaceae/Labiatae
Cautions: Use in small doses, Pregnancy
Coriander MW (Bi/expel wind damp cold, Nourish yin/liver, Spleen qi, Tonify qi/kidney, Wei qi) Apiaceae/Umbelliferae
Cautions: Pregnancy, Can be photosensitive
Fennel MW (Drain damp, Nourish yin, Spleen qi, Tonify qi/lung, Tonify yang) Apiaceae/Umbelliferae
Cautions: Estrogenic, Heat, Interior wind, Pregnancy, Cancer, Hypothyroidism
Middle Neutral..
Geranium T/MN (Astringe/lower, Calm the shen, Cool the blood, Food stasis, Nourish yin, Parasites, Smooth liver qi, Spleen qi, Tonify qi/kidney, Other: Regulates menses) Gereniaceae
Cautions: Estrogenic, Pregnancy

Middle Cooling..

Carrot (seed) MC (Drain damp, Nourish blood, Nourish yin/liver, Smooth liver qi) Apiaceae/Umbelliferae

Celery Seed MC (Bi/wind damp, Clear fire toxin, Drain damp, Food stasis, Nourish yin/liver, Regulate qi, Smooth liver qi, Spleen qi, Tonify qi/kidney) Apiaceae/Umbelliferae
Cautions: Estrogenic, Photosensitive, Pregnancy, Breastfeeding

Clary Sage MC (Clear heat/stomach, Cool the blood, Nourish yin, Smooth liver qi, Spleen qi, Subdue wind, Tonify qi/heart/lung, Other: Clear empty heat, Encourages labor, Regulates menses, Running piglet qi) Lamiaceae/Labiatae
Cautions: Estrogenic, Can be narcotic in larger doses, Cancer, Pregnancy, Alcohol consumption

German Chamomile MC (Calm the shen, Clear heat/liver/stomach/heart, Drain Damp, Nourish yin/heart, Smoothes Liver Qi, Spleen qi, Subdue wind, Tonify qi/Lung) Asteraceae/Compositae

Lavender T/MC (Calm the Shen, Clear heat/lung/liver, Nourish yin, Parasites, Regulate qi, Release the exterior, Smooth liver qi, Tonify qi/heart, Tonify yang/heart, Other: Diffuse lung qi) Lamiaceae/Labiatae

Roman Chamomille MC (Calm the Shen, Clear heat/liver, Nourish blood, Nourish yin/liver, Regulate qi, Smooth liver qi, Subdue wind) Asteraceae/Compositae
Cautions: Yang deficiency, Ragweed allergy

Sage T/MC (Clear heat/stomach, Nourish yin, Release exterior, Resolve phlegm, Tonifies Qi/kidney, Other: Promote bile, Wei qi) Lamiaceae/Labiatae
Cautions: May be estrogenic, Seizures, Pregnancy, Tisserand recommends avoiding Sage in aromatherapy.

Ylang Ylang M/BC (Calm the Shen, Clear heat/heart fire, Cool the blood, Nourish yin/heart/kidney, Tonifies qi/kidney, Wei qi) Annonaceae
Cautions: Yang deficiency, Cold

Base Warming..

Valerian BW (Nourish blood, Nourish yin, Parasites, Regulate Qi, Subdue wind, Tonifies Qi/heart, Tonify Yang/heart, Wei qi) Valerianaceae
Cautions: Qi deficiency, Yang deficiency, Pregnancy, Children

Base Neutral..

Rose BN (Clear heat/liver, Cool the blood, Invigorate blood, Nourish yin, Open orifice, Smooth liver qi, Other: Harmonize kidney/heart, Promote bile) Roseaceae

Base Cooling..

Jasmine BC (Clear heat/Liver, Nourish yin, Other: Clear empty heat, Promote childbirth) Oleaceae
Cautions: Yang deficiency

Oakmoss BC (Nourish yin/lung, Resolve phlegm) Usneaceae
Caution: Can be sensitizing, Epilepsy, Toxicity, Pregnancy
Sandalwood BsC (Calm the Shen, Clear heat/Lower Jiao, Dry damp, Nourish yin, Moves qi and blood,Other: Opens diaphragm) Santalaceae
Spikenard BC (Calms the shen, Clear heat/Heart, Nourish yin/heart, Smooths liver qi, Subdue wind) Valerianaceae
Cautions: Exogenous conditions
Vetiver BC (Calm the Shen, Clear heat, Cool the blood, Invigorate blood, Nourish blood, Nourish yin, Smooth liver qi, Spleen qi, Tonify qi/heart) Gramineae
Ylang Ylang M/BC (Calm the Shen, Clear heat/heart fire, Cool the blood, Nourish yin/heart/kidney, Tonifies qi/kidney, Wei qi) Annonaceae
Cautions: Yang deficiency, Cold

OPEN ORIFICE

Top Warming..
Camphor THot (Bi/expel wind damp, Invigorate blood, Open orifice, Parasites, Resolve phlegm) Lauraceae
Cautions: Pregnancy, Epilepsy, Can irritate mucous membranes, Toxicity
Top Cooling..
Peppermint T/MC (Clear heat, Open portals, Regulate qi, Release exterior, Smooth liver qi, Spleen qi, Tonify qi/lung, Other: Move wei qi, Relieve itch)Lamiaceae/Labiatae
Cautions: Young children, Cardiac fibrillation, Epilepsy, Mucous membranes, Neurotoxic
Middle Warming..
Oregano MW (Bi/expel wind damp cold, Move qi and blood, Open orifice, Parasites, Spleen qi, Wei qi, Other: Promotes menstruation) Lamiaceae/Labiatae
Cautions: Heat/empty heat, Pregnancy, Liver toxicity
Middle Cooling..
Peppermint T/MC (Clear heat, Open portals, Regulate qi, Release exterior, Smooth liver qi, Spleen qi, Tonify qi/lung, Other: Move wei qi, Relieve itch) Lamiaceae/Labiatae
Cautions: Young children, Cardiac fibrillation, Epilepsy, Mucous membranes, Neurotoxic
Base Warming..
Styrax BW (Bi/expel wind damp cold, Food stasis, Invigorate blood, Open portals, Parasites, Resolve phlegm/turbid, Other: Promote menstruation) Styracaceae
Cautions: Pregnancy, Yang collapse, High fever
Base Neutral..
Rose BN (Clear heat/liver, Cool the blood, Invigorate blood, Nourish yin, Open orifice, Smooth liver qi, Other: Harmonize kidney/heart, Promote bile) Roseaceae
Base Cooling..
Atlas Cedar BC (Open orifice, Resolve phlegm, Smooth liver qi) Coniferae
Cautions: Prepubescent children, Pregnancy

PARASITES

Top Warming..
Ajowan Seed TW (Parasites, Spleen qi, Tonifies Qi/Lung, Tonify Yang, Wei qi)
Cautions: Pregnancy
Camphor THot (Bi/expel wind damp, Invigorate blood, Open orifice, Parasites, Resolve phlegm) Lauraceae
Cautions: Pregnancy, Epilepsy, Can irritate mucous membranes, Toxicity
Clove THot (Parasites, Spleen qi, Tonify yang/kidney, Warm interior to expel cold) Myrtaceae
Cautions: Yin deficiency, Pregnancy, May prevent coagulation
Eucalyptus Globulus T/MW (Drain damp, Move qi and blood, Parasites, Release the exterior, Wei qi) Myrtaceae
Cautions: Children and babies
Top Neutral..
Geranium T/MN (Astringe/lower, Calm the shen, Cool the blood, Food stasis, Nourish yin, Parasites, Smooth liver qi, Spleen qi, Tonify qi/kidney, Other: Regulates menses) Gereniaceae
Cautions: Estrogenic, Pregnancy
Top Cooling..
Lavender T/MC (Calm the Shen, Clear heat/lung/liver, Nourish yin, Parasites, Regulate qi, Release the exterior, Smooth liver qi, Tonify qi/heart, Tonify yang/heart, Other: Diffuse lung qi) Lamiaceae/Labiatae
Middle Warming..
Eucalyptus Globulus T/MW (Drain damp, Move qi and blood, Parasites, Release the exterior, Wei qi) Myrtaceae
Cautions: Children and babies
Garlic MW (Parasites, Other: Detoxify) Liliaceae, Amaryllidaceae
Cautions: Heat/empty heat, Yin deficiency
Ginger M/BHot (Invigorate blood, Parasites, Release exterior, Spleen qi, Tonify qi/lung/heart/kidney, Tonify yang, Warm interior to expel cold, Wei qi, Other: Harmonize blends) Zingiberaceae
Cautions: Heat/empty heat, Stomach fire
Onion MW (Invigorate blood, Parasites, Resolve phlegm, Warm interior to expel cold) Liliaceae
Cautions: Heat/empty heat
Oregano MW (Bi/expel wind damp cold, Move qi and blood, Open orifice, Parasites, Spleen qi, Wei qi, Other: Promotes menstruation) Lamiaceae/Labiatae
Cautions: Heat/empty heat, Pregnancy, Liver toxicity

Savory MW (Nourish blood, Parasites, Resolve phlegm, Spleen qi, Tonify qi) Lamiaceae/Labiatae
Cautions: Heat/empty heat, Pregnancy
Tarragon MW (Food stasis, Moves qi and blood, Nourish Blood, Parasites, Spleen qi, Tonify Qi/heart, Other: Promote menstruation) Asteraceae
Cautions: Pregnancy, Cancer

Middle Neutral...

Geranium T/MN (Astringe/lower, Calm the shen, Cool the blood, Food stasis, Nourish yin, Parasites, Smooth liver qi, Spleen qi, Tonify qi/kidney, Other: Regulates menses) Gereniaceae
Cautions: Estrogenic, Pregnancy
Rosewood MN (Parasites, Regulate qi, Release the exterior, Smooth liver qi, Spleen qi, Tonify qi, Wei qi) Lauraceae

Middle Cooling...

Cajeput MC (Bi/Expel damp hot, Drain damp/lower jiao, Move qi and blood, Parasites, Release exterior, Tonify qi/lung) Myrtaceae
Lavender T/MC (Calm the Shen, Clear heat/lung/liver, Nourish yin, Parasites, Regulate qi, Release the exterior, Smooth liver qi, Tonify qi/heart, Tonify yang/heart, Other: Diffuse lung qi) Lamiaceae/Labiatae
Melissa MC (Astringe/blood, Clear heat/liver/heart/wei, Cools the blood, Food stasis, Parasites, Regulate qi, Release the exterior, Smooth liver qi, Other: Open and relax the chest) Lamiaceae/Labiatae
Cautions: Can be sensitizing in high doses.
Niaouli MC (Bi/wind damp/lower, Invigorate blood, Parasites, Release the exterior, Spleen qi, Tonify qi/lung/kidney, Wei qi) Myrtaceae
Cautions: Pregnancy, Children
Tea Tree MC (Clear heat, Dry damp, Invigorate blood, Parasites, Release exterior, Tonify qi, Wei qi) Myraceae
Thyme Linalool MC (Clear heat/lung/stomach, Parasites, Tonify qi) Lamiaceae/Labiatae
Cautions: Glaucoma

Base Warming..

Balsam of Peru BW (Calm the Shen, Moves qi and blood, Parasites, Resolve phlegm, Tonifies Qi/Heart, Wei qi) Fabaceae
Cautions: May cause sensitization, Pregnancy, Breastfeeding
Cinnamon BHot (Astringe/blood, Bi/expel wind damp, Drain damp, Invigorate blood, Nourish blood, Parasites, Spleen qi, Tonify qi, Tonify yang, Warm interior to expel cold, Wei qi, Other: Regulate menstruation) Lauraceae
Cautions: Heat/empty heat, Mucous membranes, Pregnancy, May sensitize skin, Kidney, Liver toxicity, May prevent coagulation

Ginger M/BHot (Invigorate blood, Parasites, Release exterior, Spleen qi, Tonify qi/lung/heart/kidney, Tonify yang, Warm interior to expel cold, Wei qi, Other: Harmonize blends) Zingiberaceae
Cautions: Heat/empty heat, Stomach fire
Styrax BW (Bi/expel wind damp cold, Food stasis, Invigorate blood, Open portals, Parasites, Resolve phlegm/turbid, Other: Promote menstruation) Styracaceae
Cautions: Pregnancy, Yang collapse, High fever
Valerian BW (Nourish blood, Nourish yin, Parasites, Regulate Qi, Subdue wind, Tonifies Qi/heart, Tonify Yang/heart, Wei qi) Valerianaceae
Cautions: Qi deficiency, Yang deficiency, Pregnancy, Children

REGULATE QI

Top Warming...
Eucalyptus Globulus T/MW (Drain damp, Move qi and blood, Parasites, Release the exterior, Wei qi) Myrtaceae
Cautions: Children and babies
Grapefruit TsWd (Drain damp, Food stasis, Regulate qi, Resolve phlegm, Smooth liver qi, Other, Promote bile production) Rutaceae
Cautions: Photosensitive, Heat patterns
Rosemary T/MW (Nourish blood, Regulate qi, Release the exterior, Spleen qi, Tonify qi/kidney/heart, Tonify yang, Warm the interior to expel cold) Lamiaceae/Labiatae
Cautions: Heat/empty heat, Pregnancy, Children, Rebellious qi, Hypertension
Top Cooling...
Bay Laurel TsC (Food stasis, Regulate qi/stomach, Resolve hot phlegm) Lauraceae
Cautions: Narcotic in large doses, Pregnancy
Bergamot T/MsC (Clear heat/fire toxin, Drain damp, Food stagnation, Regulate qi, Release exterior, Smooth liver qi, Wei qi) Rutacae
Cautions: Photosensitive
Bitter Orange TCold (Food stagnation, Regulate qi/liver/stomach, Smooth liver qi, Spleen qi) Rutacae
Cautions: Photosensitive, Qi deficiency, Cold stomach
Blue Yarrow TC (Clear Heat, Moves qi and blood, Tonifies qi/heart)
Cautions: Pregnancy
Eucalyptus Citriodora TC (Drain damp, Move qi and blood, Wei qi,) Myrtaceae
Cautions: Children
Lavender T/MC (Calm the Shen, Clear heat/lung/liver, Nourish yin, Parasites, Regulate qi, Release the exterior, Smooth liver qi, Tonify qi/heart, Tonify yang/heart, Other: Diffuse lung qi) Lamiaceae/Labiatae
Lime TC (Regulate qi/stomach/spleen, Wei qi, Other: Uplift mood) Rutaceae
Cautions: Photosensitive
Mandarin TC (Calm the Shen, Food stasis, Regulate qi, Spleen qi, Subdue wind) Rutaceae
Orange TC (Clear heat/Heart, Food stasis, Regulate qi, Release exterior, Smooth liver qi, Spleen qi, Other: Clear heart fire) Rutaceae
Caution: Photosensitive

Peppermint T/MC (Clear heat, Open portals, Regulate qi, Release exterior, Smooth liver qi, Spleen qi, Tonify qi/lung, Other: Move wei qi, Relieve itch) Lamiaceae/Labiatae
Cautions: Young children, Cardiac fibrillation, Epilepsy, Mucous membranes, Neurotoxic
Petitgrain T/MC (Calm the shen, Drain damp, Regulate qi/chest, Smooth liver qi) Rutaceae
Sweet Marjoram T/MC (Bi/expel damp hot, Clear heat/liver, Food stasis, Regulate qi, Release exterior, Smooth liver qi, Stop coughing) Lamiaceae/Labiatae
Cautions: Asthma, Pregnancy
Tangerine TC (Nourish blood, Move qi and blood, Spleen qi) Rutaceae
Cautions: May be photosensitive
Middle Warming...

Cardamom MW (Food stasis, Invigorate blood, Regulate qi, Spleen qi, Stop coughing, Tonify qi/Lung) Zingiberaceae
Cautions: Yin deficiency, Blood deficiency
Eucalyptus Globulus T/MW (Drain damp, Move qi and blood, Parasites, Release the exterior, Wei qi) Myrtaceae
Cautions: Children and babies
Litsea MW (Bi/expel wind damp cold, Invigorate blood/lower, Regulate qi/lower, Release the exterior, Spleen qi, Tonify yang) Lauraceae
Cautions: Yin deficiency with heat
Nutmeg MW (Nourish blood, Move qi and blood, Spleen qi, Tonify yang/spleen/kidney, Warm interior to expel cold) Myristicaceae
Cautions: Diarrhea due to heat, Liver wind/ascending yang, Epilepsy, Liver toxicity, Pregnancy, High doses can produce delirium convulsions, Hallucinations, Dizziness, Fainting, Cancer
Oregano MW (Bi/expel wind damp cold, Move qi and blood, Open orifice, Parasites, Spleen qi, Wei qi, Other: Promotes menstruation) Lamiaceae/Labiatae
Cautions: Heat/empty heat, Pregnancy, Liver toxicity
Parsley MW (Drain damp/lower, Invigorate blood, Regulate qi/stomach, Other: Abortion, Childbirth, Promote menstruation) Umbelliferae
Cautions: Neurotoxic, Liver toxic, Pregnancy, Breastfeeding
Rosemary T/MW (Nourish blood, Regulate qi, Release the exterior, Spleen qi, Tonify qi/kidney/heart, Tonify yang, Warm the interior to expel cold) Lamiaceae/Labiatae
Cautions: Heat/empty heat, Pregnancy, Children, Rebellious qi, Hypertension
Tarragon MW (Food stasis, Moves qi and blood, Nourish Blood, Parasites, Spleen qi, Tonify Qi/heart, Other: Promote menstruation) Asteraceae
Cautions: Pregnancy, Cancer

Middle Neutral...

Rosewood MN (Parasites, Regulate qi, Release the exterior, Smooth liver qi, Spleen qi, Tonify qi, Wei qi) Lauraceae

Middle Cooling...

Anise MC (Clear heat, Food stagnation, Regulate qi, Smooth liver qi, Stop cough, Other: Promote lactation) Apiaceae/Umbelliferae
Cautions: Mild estrogenic, Yin deficiency, Cancer, Pregnancy

Bergamot T/MsC (Clear heat/fire toxin, Drain damp, Food stagnation, Regulate qi, Release exterior, Smooth liver qi, Wei qi) Rutacae
Cautions: Photosensitive

Cajeput MC (Bi/Expel damp hot, Drain damp/lower jiao, Move qi and blood, Parasites, Release exterior, Tonify qi/lung) Myrtaceae

Celery Seed MC (Bi/wind damp, Clear fire toxin, Drain damp, Food stasis, Nourish yin/liver, Regulate qi, Smooth liver qi, Spleen qi, Tonify qi/kidney) Apiaceae/Umbelliferae
Cautions: Estrogenic, Photosensitive, Pregnancy, Breastfeeding

Cypress M/BsC (Astringe, Clear heat/lung, Move qi and blood, Stop coughing, Other: Ascend spleen qi, Assist kidney to grasp lung qi) Cupressaceae
Cautions: Hypertension, Cancer

Lavender T/MC (Calm the Shen, Clear heat/lung/liver, Nourish yin, Parasites, Regulate qi, Release the exterior, Smooth liver qi, Tonify qi/heart, Tonify yang/heart, Other: Diffuse lung qi) Lamiaceae/Labiatae

Melissa MC (Astringe/blood, Clear heat/liver/heart/wei, Cools the blood, Food stasis, Parasites, Regulate qi, Release the exterior, Smooth liver qi, Other: Open and relax the chest) Lamiaceae/Labiatae
Cautions: Can be sensitizing in high doses.

Peppermint T/MC (Clear heat, Open portals, Regulate qi, Release exterior, Smooth liver qi, Spleen qi, Tonify qi/lung, Other: Move wei qi, Relieve itch) Lamiaceae/Labiatae
Cautions: Young children, Cardiac fibrillation, Epilepsy, Mucous membranes, Neurotoxic

Petitgrain T/MC (Calm the shen, Drain damp, Regulate qi/chest, Smooth liver qi) Rutaceae

Roman Chamomille MC (Calm the Shen, Clear heat/liver, Nourish blood, Nourish yin/liver, Regulate qi, Smooth liver qi, Subdue wind) Asteraceae/Compositae
Cautions: Yang deficiency, Ragweed allergy

Sweet Marjoram T/MC (Bi/expel damp hot, Clear heat/liver, Food stasis, Regulate qi, Release exterior, Smooth liver qi, Stop coughing) Lamiaceae/Labiatae
Cautions: Asthma, Pregnancy

Yarrow MCold (Clear heat, Moves qi and blood, Smoothes liver qi, Spleen qi, Tonifies qi/heart/kidney, Other: Ascend spleen qi, Promote sweating) Asteracea/Compositae
Cautions: Neurotoxic, Children, Pregnancy, Ragweed allergy
Base Warming...

Balsam of Peru BW (Calm the Shen, Moves qi and blood, Parasites, Resolve phlegm, Tonifies Qi/Heart, Wei qi) Fabaceae
Cautions: May cause sensitization, Pregnancy, Breastfeeding
Elemi BWd (Invigorate blood/chest, Regulate qi/chest, Resolve phlegm) Berseraceae
Cautions: Pregnancy
Valerian BW (Nourish blood, Nourish yin, Parasites, Regulate Qi, Subdue wind, Tonifies Qi/heart, Tonify Yang/heart, Wei qi) Valerianaceae
Cautions: Qi deficiency, Yang deficiency, Pregnancy, Children
Base Cooling...

Cypress M/BsC (Astringe, Clear heat/lung, Move qi and blood, Stop coughing, Other: Ascend spleen qi, Assist kidney to grasp lung qi) Cupressaceae
Cautions: Hypertension, Cancer
Frankincense BsCd (Calm the shen, Clear heat/Lung/Stomach, Dry damp, Nourish blood/liver, Resolve phlegm, Strongly move qi and blood, Tonify qi/lung, Other: Reduce swelling) Berceraceae
Cautions: Pregnancy
Helichrysum BC (Bi/expel damp hot, Clear heat/Lung/Liver/Fire Toxin, Cool the blood, Move qi and blood, Nourish blood, Smooth liver qi, Wei qi) Asteracea/Compositae
Cautions: Yang deficiency
Myrrh BC (Clear heat/Lung/Stomach, Dry damp, Move qi and blood, Spleen qi, Other: Promotes healing of wounds) Burseraceae
Cautions: Pregnancy, Uterine bleeding
Sandalwood BsC (Calm the Shen, Clear heat/Lower Jiao, Dry damp, Nourish yin, Moves qi and blood, Other: Opens diaphragm) Santalaceae

RELEASE THE EXTERIOR

Top Warming..
Basil T/MW (Food stasis, Nourish yin/liver, Release the exterior, Spleen qi, Tonify qi//kidney, Tonify yang, Wei qi, Other: Promote lactation, Relieve uterine contraction) Lamiaceae/Labiatae
Cautions: Use in small doses, Pregnancy
Eucalyptus Globulus T/MW (Drain damp, Move qi and blood, Parasites, Release the exterior, Wei qi) Myrtaceae
Cautions: Children and babies
Rosemary T/MW (Nourish blood, Regulate qi, Release the exterior, Spleen qi, Tonify qi/kidney/heart, Tonify yang, Warm the interior to expel cold) Lamiaceae/Labiatae
Cautions: Heat/empty heat, Pregnancy, Children, Rebellious qi, Hypertension
Top Cooling..
Bergamot T/MsC (Clear heat/fire toxin, Drain damp, Food stagnation, Regulate qi, Release exterior, Smooth liver qi, Wei qi) Rutacae
Cautions: Photosensitive
Citronella TCold (Release the exterior, Tonify qi, Wei qi) Graminae
Cautions: Yang deficiency
Lavender T/MC (Calm the Shen, Clear heat/lung/liver, Nourish yin, Parasites, Regulate qi, Release the exterior, Smooth liver qi, Tonify qi/heart, Tonify yang/heart, Other: Diffuse lung qi) Lamiaceae/Labiatae
Orange TC (Clear heat/Heart, Food stasis, Regulate qi, Release exterior, Smooth liver qi, Spleen qi, Other: Clear heart fire) Rutaceae
Caution: Photosensitive
Palmarosa TC (Clear heat, Drain damp/lower, Nourish yin, Release the exterior, Smooth liver qi, Other: Clear damp heat skin outbreaks) Poaceae
Peppermint T/MC (Clear heat, Open portals, Regulate qi, Release exterior, Smooth liver qi, Spleen qi, Tonify qi/lung, Other: Move wei qi, Relieve itch) Lamiaceae/Labiatae
Cautions: Young children, Cardiac fibrillation, Epilepsy, Mucous membranes, Neurotoxic
Rosalina TC (Clear heat/stomach, Release the exterior) Myrtaceae
Caution: Pregnancy
Sage T/MC (Clear heat/stomach, Nourish yin, Release exterior, Resolve phlegm, Tonifies Qi/kidney, Other: Promote bile, Wei qi) Lamiaceae/Labiatae
Cautions: May be estrogenic, Seizures, Pregnancy, Tisserand recommends avoiding Sage in aromatherapy.

Spearmint T/MC (Calm the shen, Release the exterior, Smooth liver qi, Spleen qi, Wei qi, Other: Relieve itch) Lamiaceae/Labiatae
Cautions: Neurotoxic, Pregnancy, Mucous membranes
Sweet Marjoram T/MC (Bi/expel damp hot, Clear heat/liver, Food stasis, Regulate qi, Release exterior, Smooth liver qi, Stop coughing) Lamiaceae/Labiatae
Cautions: Asthma, Pregnancy
Middle Warming...
Basil T/MW (Food stasis, Nourish yin/liver, Release the exterior, Spleen qi, Tonify qi//kidney, Tonify yang, Wei qi, Other: Promote lactation, Relieve uterine contraction) Lamiaceae/Labiatae
Cautions: Use in small doses, Pregnancy
Birch MW (Bi/expel wind damp cold, Clear Heat, Drain damp, Release exterior, Other: Open joints) Betulaceae
Cautions: Kidney toxicity, Kidney deficiency, May thin the blood, Pregnancy, Breastfeeding
Black Pepper MHot (Release exterior, Spleen qi, Tonify qi/kidney, Tonify yang, Wei qi) Piperacea
Cautions: Deficiency heat, Pregnancy
Cinnamon Leaf MW (Invigorate blood, Release exterior, Spleen qi, Other: Promote sweating, Stimulate childbirth) Lauraceae
Cautions: Heat/empty heat
Eucalyptus Globulus T/MW (Drain damp, Move qi and blood, Parasites, Release the exterior, Wei qi) Myrtaceae
Cautions: Children and babies
Ginger M/BHot (Invigorate blood, Parasites, Release exterior, Spleen qi, Tonify qi/lung/heart/kidney, Tonify yang, Warm interior to expel cold, Wei qi, Other: Harmonize blends) Zingiberaceae
Cautions: Heat/empty heat, Stomach fire
Litsea MW (Bi/expel wind damp cold, Invigorate blood/lower, Regulate qi/lower, Release the exterior, Spleen qi, Tonify yang) Lauraceae
Cautions: Yin deficiency with heat
Pine MW (Release the exterior, Resolve phlegm, Spleen qi, Stop cough, Tonify qi/lung/kidney, Tonify yang, Other: Descend qi to kidneys) Pinaceae
Cautions: Yin deficiency, Blood deficiency
Rosemary T/MW (Nourish blood, Regulate qi, Release the exterior, Spleen qi, Tonify qi/kidney/heart, Tonify yang, Warm the interior to expel cold) Lamiaceae/Labiatae
Cautions: Heat/empty heat, Pregnancy, Children, Rebellious qi, Hypertension

Terebinth MW (Bi/expel wind damp cold, Release Exterior, Subdue wind) Pinaceae
Cautions: Yin deficiency/liver/kidney, Blood deficiency, Epilepsy
Wintergreen MW (Bi/expel wind damp hot, Release the exterior, Smooth liver qi) Ericaceae
Cautions: Kidney toxicity in overuse, Pregnancy
Middle Neutral...
Rosewood MN (Parasites, Regulate qi, Release the exterior, Smooth liver qi, Spleen qi, Tonify qi, Wei qi) Lauraceae
Middle Cooling...
Bergamot T/MsC (Clear heat/fire toxin, Drain damp, Food stagnation, Regulate qi, Release exterior, Smooth liver qi, Wei qi) Rutacae
Cautions: Photosensitive
Cajeput MC (Bi/Expel damp hot, Drain damp/lower jiao, Move qi and blood, Parasites, Release exterior, Tonify qi/lung) Myrtaceae
Ho Leaf MC (Release exterior, Resolve phlegm, Spleen qi, Other: Harmonize Blends) Lauraceae
Cautions: Yang deficiency
Lavender T/MC (Calm the Shen, Clear heat/lung/liver, Nourish yin, Parasites, Regulate qi, Release the exterior, Smooth liver qi, Tonify qi/heart, Tonify yang/heart, Other: Diffuse lung qi) Lamiaceae/Labiatae
Melissa MC (Astringe/blood, Clear heat/liver/heart/wei, Cools the blood, Food stasis, Parasites, Regulate qi, Release the exterior, Smooth liver qi, Other: Open and relax the chest) Lamiaceae/Labiatae
Cautions: Can be sensitizing in high doses.
Niaouli MC (Bi/wind damp/lower, Invigorate blood, Parasites, Release the exterior, Spleen qi, Tonify qi/lung/kidney, Wei qi) Myrtaceae
Cautions: Pregnancy, Children
Peppermint T/MC (Clear heat, Open portals, Regulate qi, Release exterior, Smooth liver qi, Spleen qi, Tonify qi/lung, Other: Move wei qi, Relieve itch) Lamiaceae/Labiatae
Cautions: Young children, Cardiac fibrillation, Epilepsy, Mucous membranes, Neurotoxic
Ravensare MC (Clear heat/lung, Release exterior) Lauraceae
Sage TMC (Clear heat/stomach, Nourish yin, Release exterior, Resolve phlegm, Tonifies Qi/kidney, Other: Promote bile, Wei qi) Lamiaceae/Labiatae
Cautions: May be estrogenic, Seizures, Pregnancy, Tisserand recommends avoiding Sage in aromatherapy.
Spearmint T/MC (Calm the shen, Release the exterior, Smooth liver qi, Spleen qi, Wei qi, Other: Relieve itch) Lamiaceae/Labiatae
Cautions: Neurotoxic, Pregnancy, Mucous membranes

Sweet Marjoram T/MC (Bi/expel damp hot, Clear heat/liver, Food stasis, Regulate qi, Release exterior, Smooth liver qi, Stop coughing) Lamiaceae/Labiatae
Cautions: Asthma, Pregnancy
Tea Tree MC (Clear heat, Dry damp, Invigorate blood, Parasites, Release exterior, Tonify qi, Wei qi) Myraceae
Base Warming..
Ginger M/BHot (Invigorate blood, Parasites, Release exterior, Spleen qi, Tonify qi/lung/heart/kidney, Tonify yang, Warm interior to expel cold, Wei qi, Other: Harmonize blends) Zingiberaceae
Cautions: Heat/empty heat, Stomach fire
Patchouli BsW (Clear summer heat, Release the exterior, Strongly tonify spleen qi, Other: Release suppressed emotion) Lamiaceae/Labiatae

RESOLVE PHLEGM

Top Warming...

Camphor THot (Bi/expel wind damp, Invigorate blood, Open orifice, Parasites, Resolve phlegm) Lauraceae
Cautions: Pregnancy, Epilepsy, Can irritate mucous membranes, Toxicity

Eucalyptus Radiata TW (Drain damp, Resolve Phlegm, Tonify qi, Wei qi) Myrtaceae

Grapefruit TsWd (Drain damp, Food stasis, Regulate qi, Resolve phlegm, Smooth liver qi, Other, Promote bile production) Rutaceae
Cautions: Photosensitive, Heat patterns

Top Cooling...

Bay Laurel TsC (Food stasis, Regulate qi/stomach, Resolve hot phlegm) Lauraceae
Cautions: Narcotic in large doses, Pregnancy

Eucalyptus Smithii TC (Drain damp, Resolve Phlegm, Tonifies Qi, Wei qi) Myrtaceae
Cautions: Children 3 and under, Pregnancy

Sage T/MC (Clear heat/stomach, Nourish yin, Release exterior, Resolve phlegm, Tonifies Qi/kidney, Other: Promote bile, Wei qi) Lamiaceae/Labiatae
Cautions: May be estrogenic, Seizures, Pregnancy, Tisserand recommends avoiding Sage in aromatherapy.

Middle Warming...

Caraway MW (Resolve damp phlegm, Spleen qi, Tonify qi, Other: Descend qi) Apiaceae/Umbelliferae Cautions: Pregnancy, Children under 3, Cancer

Juniper MW (Drain damp, Invigorate blood, Resolve phlegm, Spleen qi, Tonify yang/strongly, Other: Promote menstruation) Cupressaceae
Cautions: Kidney yin deficiency, Kidney toxicity, Pregnancy

Onion MW (Invigorate blood, Parasites, Resolve phlegm, Warm interior to expel cold) Liliaceae
Cautions: Heat/empty heat

Pine MW (Release the exterior, Resolve phlegm, Spleen qi, Stop cough, Tonify qi/lung/kidney, Tonify yang, Other: Descend qi to kidneys) Pinaceae
Cautions: Yin deficiency, Blood deficiency

Savory MW (Nourish blood, Parasites, Resolve phlegm, Spleen qi, Tonify qi) Lamiaceae/Labiatae
Cautions: Heat/empty heat, Pregnancy

Middle Cooling...

Fir MC (Bi/expel damp hot, Clear heat, Dry damp/lower, Resolve phlegm/damp, Stop coughing, Tonify qi/lung, Other: Help kidneys grasp qi) Pinaceae

Ho Leaf MC (Release exterior, Resolve phlegm, Spleen qi, Other: Harmonize Blends) Lauraceae
Cautions: Yang deficiency

Sage T/MC (Clear heat/stomach, Nourish yin, Release exterior, Resolve phlegm, Tonifies Qi/kidney, Other: Promote bile, Wei qi) Lamiaceae/Labiatae
Cautions: May be estrogenic, Seizures, Pregnancy, Tisserand recommends avoiding Sage in aromatherapy.

Base Warming...

Balsam of Peru BW (Calm the Shen, Moves qi and blood, Parasites, Resolve phlegm, Tonifies Qi/Heart, Wei qi) Fabaceae
Cautions: May cause sensitization, Pregnancy, Breastfeeding

Elemi BWd (Invigorate blood/chest, Regulate qi/chest, Resolve phlegm) Berseraceae
Cautions: Pregnancy

Styrax BW (Bi/expel wind damp cold, Food stasis, Invigorate blood, Open portals, Parasites, Resolve phlegm/turbid, Other: Promote menstruation) Styracaceae
Cautions: Pregnancy, Yang collapse, High fever

Base Cooling...

Atlas Cedar BC (Open orifice, Resolve phlegm, Smooth liver qi) Coniferae
Cautions: Prepubescent children, Pregnancy

Frankincense BsCd (Calm the shen, Clear heat/Lung/Stomach, Dry damp, Nourish blood/liver, Resolve phlegm, Strongly move qi and blood, Tonify qi/lung, Other: Reduce swelling) Berceraceae
Cautions: Pregnancy

Lovage BCold (Clear heat/stomach/kidney, Drain damp, Resolve phlegm, Spleen qi) Apiaceae/Umbelliferae
Cautions: Photosensitive, Toxic

Marigold BC (Clear heat, Resolve hot phlegm, Other: Promote bile secretion) Asteracea/Compositae
Cautions: Photosensitive, Toxic, Epilepsy, Pregnancy

Oakmoss BC (Nourish yin/lung, Resolve phlegm) Usneaceae
Caution: Can be sensitizing, Epilepsy, Toxicity, Pregnancy

SMOOTH LIVER QI

Top Warming..
Grapefruit TsWd (Drain damp, Food stasis, Regulate qi, Resolve phlegm, Smooth liver qi, Other, Promote bile production) Rutaceae
Cautions: Photosensitive, Heat patterns

Top Neutral..
Geranium T/MN (Astringe/lower, Calm the shen, Cool the blood, Food stasis, Nourish yin, Parasites, Smooth liver qi, Spleen qi, Tonify qi/kidney, Other: Regulates menses) Gereniaceae
Cautions: Estrogenic, Pregnancy

Top Cooling..
Bergamot T/MsC (Clear heat/fire toxin, Drain damp, Food stagnation, Regulate qi, Release exterior, Smooth liver qi, Wei qi) Rutacae
Cautions: Photosensitive

Bitter Orange TCold (Food stagnation, Regulate qi/liver/stomach, Smooth liver qi, Spleen qi) Rutacae
Cautions: Photosensitive, Qi deficiency, Cold stomach

Lavender T/MC (Calm the Shen, Clear heat/lung/liver, Nourish yin, Parasites, Regulate qi, Release the exterior, Smooth liver qi, Tonify qi/heart, Tonify yang/heart, Other: Diffuse lung qi) Lamiaceae/Labiatae

Lemon Verbena TC (Clear heat/Heart/Liver, Smooth liver qi) Lamiaceae/Labiatae
Cautions: Mildly photosensitive

Orange TC (Clear heat/Heart, Food stasis, Regulate qi, Release exterior, Smooth liver qi, Spleen qi, Other: Clear heart fire) Rutaceae
Caution: Photosensitive

Palmarosa TC (Clear heat, Drain damp/lower, Nourish yin, Release the exterior, Smooth liver qi, Other: Clear damp heat skin outbreaks) Poaceae

Peppermint T/MC (Clear heat, Open portals, Regulate qi, Release exterior, Smooth liver qi, Spleen qi, Tonify qi/lung, Other: Move wei qi, Relieve itch) Lamiaceae/Labiatae
Cautions: Young children, Cardiac fibrillation, Epilepsy, Mucous membranes, Neurotoxic

Petitgrain T/MC (Calm the shen, Drain damp, Regulate qi/chest, Smooth liver qi) Rutaceae

Spearmint T/MC (Calm the shen, Release the exterior, Smooth liver qi, Spleen qi, Wei qi, Other: Relieve itch) Lamiaceae/Labiatae
Cautions: Neurotoxic, Pregnancy, Mucous membranes

Sweet Marjoram T/MC (Bi/expel damp hot, Clear heat/liver, Food stasis, Regulate qi, Release exterior, Smooth liver qi, Stop coughing) Lamiaceae/Labiatae
Cautions: Asthma, Pregnancy
Middle Warming..

Cumin MsW (Invigorate blood, Smooth liver qi, Spleen qi, Tonify qi/heart) Apiaceae/Umbelliferae
Cautions: Photosensitive, Pregnancy

Wintergreen MW (Bi/expel wind damp hot, Release the exterior, Smooth liver qi) Ericaceae
Cautions: Kidney toxicity in overuse, Pregnancy
Middle Neutral...

Geranium T/MN (Astringe/lower, Calm the shen, Cool the blood, Food stasis, Nourish yin, Parasites, Smooth liver qi, Spleen qi, Tonify qi/kidney, Other: Regulates menses) Gereniaceae
Cautions: Estrogenic, Pregnancy

Rosewood MN (Parasites, Regulate qi, Release the exterior, Smooth liver qi, Spleen qi, Tonify qi, Wei qi) Lauraceae
Middle Coooling...

Anise MC (Clear heat, Food stagnation, Regulate qi, Smooth liver qi, Stop cough, Other: Promote lactation) Apiaceae/Umbelliferae
Cautions: Mild estrogenic, Yin deficiency, Cancer, Pregnancy

Bergamot T/MsC (Clear heat/fire toxin, Drain damp, Food stagnation, Regulate qi, Release exterior, Smooth liver qi, Wei qi) Rutacae
Cautions: Photosensitive

Carrot (seed) MC (Drain damp, Nourish blood, Nourish yin/liver, Smooth liver qi) Apiaceae/Umbelliferae

Celery Seed MC (Bi/wind damp, Clear fire toxin, Drain damp, Food stasis, Nourish yin/liver, Regulate qi, Smooth liver qi, Spleen qi, Tonify qi/kidney) Apiaceae/Umbelliferae
Cautions: Estrogenic, Photosensitive, Pregnancy, Breastfeeding

Clary Sage MC (Clear heat/stomach, Cool the blood, Nourish yin, Smooth liver qi, Spleen qi, Subdue wind, Tonify qi/heart/lung, Other: Clear empty heat, Encourages labor, Regulates menses, Running piglet qi) Lamiaceae/Labiatae
Cautions: Estrogenic, Can be narcotic in larger doses, Cancer, Pregancy, Alcohol consumption

Galbanum M/BC (Bi/expel damp hot, Calm the shen, Smooth liver qi, Tonify qi/lung,) Apiaceae/Umbelliferae

German Chamomile MC (Calm the shen, Clear heat/liver/stomach/heart, Drain Damp, Nourish yin/heart, Smoothes Liver Qi, Spleen qi, Subdue wind, Tonify qi/Lung) Asteraceae/Compositae

Lavender T/MC (Calm the Shen, Clear heat/lung/liver, Nourish yin, Parasites, Regulate qi, Release the exterior, Smooth liver qi, Tonify qi/heart, Tonify yang/heart, Other: Diffuse lung qi)
Lamiaceae/Labiatae
Lavendin MC (Clear heat/lung/liver, Smooth liver qi)Lamiaceae/Labiatae
Cautions: Yang deficiency, (Not toxic when diluted.)
Melissa MC (Astringe/blood, Clear heat/liver/heart/wei, Cools the blood, Food stasis, Parasites, Regulate qi, Release the exterior, Smooth liver qi, Other: Open and relax the chest) Lamiaceae/Labiatae
Cautions: Can be sensitizing in high doses.
Myrtle M/BCd (Astringe, Clear heat/Lung, Drain damp/lower, Smooth liver qi, Wei qi) Myrtaceae
Cautions: Yang deficiency, Cold
Peppermint T/MC (Clear heat, Open portals, Regulate qi, Release exterior, Smooth liver qi, Spleen qi, Tonify qi/lung, Other: Move wei qi, Relieve itch) Lamiaceae/Labiatae
Cautions: Young children, Cardiac fibrillation, Epilepsy, Mucous membranes, Neurotoxic
Petitgrain T/MC (Calm the shen, Drain damp, Regulate qi/chest, Smooth liver qi) Rutaceae
Roman Chamomille MC (Calm the Shen, Clear heat/liver, Nourish blood, Nourish yin/liver, Regulate qi, Smooth liver qi, Subdue wind)
Asteraceae/Compositae
Cautions: Yang deficiency, Ragweed allergy
Spearmint T/MC (Calm the shen, Release the exterior, Smooth liver qi, Spleen qi, Wei qi, Other: Relieve itch) Lamiaceae/Labiatae
Cautions: Neurotoxic, Pregnancy, Mucous membranes
Sweet Marjoram T/MC (Bi/expel damp hot, Clear heat/liver, Food stasis, Regulate qi, Release exterior, Smooth liver qi, Stop coughing)
Lamiaceae/Labiatae
Cautions: Asthma, Pregnancy
Yarrow MCold (Clear heat, Moves qi and blood, Smoothes liver qi, Spleen qi, Tonifies qi/heart/kidney, Other: Ascend spleen qi, Promote sweating)
Asteracea/Compositae
Cautions: Neurotoxic, Children, Pregnancy, Ragweed allergy
Base Warming...
Angelica BW (Calm the shen, Invigorate blood, Nourish blood, Smooth liver qi, Spleen qi, Tonify qi/lung, Wei qi, Other: Ease cough, Expel phlegm, Open the diaphragm) Apiaceae/Umbelliferae
Cautions: Photosensitive, Pregnancy, Diabetes
Cistus BsW (Smooth liver qi, Tonify spleen, Other: Stop bleeding)
Cistaceae
Cautions: Pregnancy

Base Neutral...

Rose BN (Clear heat/liver, Cool the blood, Invigorate blood, Nourish yin, Open orifice, Smooth liver qi, Other: Harmonize kidney/heart, Promote bile) Roseaceae

Base Cooling..

Atlas Cedar BC (Open orifice, Resolve phlegm, Smooth liver qi) Coniferae
Cautions: Prepubescent children, Pregnancy

Galbanum M/BC (Bi/expel damp hot, Calm the shen, Smooth liver qi, Tonify qi/lung,) Apiaceae/Umbelliferae

Helichrysum BC (Bi/expel damp hot, Clear heat/Lung/Liver/Fire Toxin, Cool the blood, Move qi and blood, Nourish blood, Smooth liver qi, Wei qi) Asteracea/Compositae
Cautions: Yang deficiency

Myrtle M/BCd (Astringe, Clear heat/Lung, Drain damp/lower, Smooth liver qi, Wei qi) Myrtaceae
Cautions: Yang deficiency, Cold

Spikenard BC (Calms the shen, Clear heat/Heart, Nourish yin/heart, Smooths liver qi, Subdue wind) Valerianaceae
Cautions: Exogenous conditions

Vetiver BC (Calm the Shen, Clear heat, Cool the blood, Invigorate blood, Nourish blood, Nourish yin, Smooth liver qi, Spleen qi, Tonify qi/heart) Gramineae

SPLEEN QI

Top Warming...
Ajowan Seed TW (Parasites, Spleen qi, Tonifies Qi/Lung, Tonify Yang, Wei qi)
Cautions: Pregnancy
Basil T/MW (Food stasis, Nourish yin/liver, Release the exterior, Spleen qi, Tonify qi//kidney, Tonify yang, Wei qi, Other: Promote lactation, Relieve uterine contraction) Lamiaceae/Labiatae
Cautions: Use in small doses, Pregnancy
Clove THot (Parasites, Spleen qi, Tonify yang/kidney, Warm interior to expel cold) Myrtaceae
Cautions: Yin deficiency, Pregnancy, May prevent coagulation
Lemongrass TW (Nourish blood, Spleen qi, Tonify yang, Warm interior to expel cold, Wei qi) Graminae
Cautions: Heat/empty heat, Glaucoma, Children, Prostatic hyperplasia, Slight risk of sensitization
Pennyroyal T/MW (Food stasis, Spleen qi, Stop coughing, Other: Promote bile, Regulate menses) Lamiaceae/Labiatae
Cautions: Pregnancy
Rosemary T/MW (Nourish blood, Regulate qi, Release the exterior, Spleen qi, Tonify qi/kidney/heart, Tonify yang, Warm the interior to expel cold) Lamiaceae/Labiatae
Cautions: Heat/empty heat, Pregnancy, Children, Rebellious qi, Hypertension
Top Neutral...
Geranium T/MN (Astringe/lower, Calm the shen, Cool the blood, Food stasis, Nourish yin, Parasites, Smooth liver qi, Spleen qi, Tonify qi/kidney, Other: Regulates menses) Gereniaceae
Cautions: Estrogenic, Pregnancy
Top Cooling...
Bitter Orange TCold (Food stagnation, Regulate qi/liver/stomach, Smooth liver qi, Spleen qi) Rutacae
Cautions: Photosensitive, Qi deficiency, Cold stomach
Lemon TCd (Bi/damp Invigorate blood, Clear heat/liver/GB/stomach, Spleen qi, Wei qi, Other: Break up stones) Rutaceae
Cautions: Photosensitive
Mandarin TC (Calm the Shen, Food stasis, Regulate qi, Spleen qi, Subdue wind) Rutaceae
Orange TC (Clear heat/Heart, Food stasis, Regulate qi, Release exterior, Smooth liver qi, Spleen qi, Other: Clear heart fire) Rutaceae
Caution: Photosensitive

Peppermint T/MC (Clear heat, Open portals, Regulate qi, Release exterior, Smooth liver qi, Spleen qi, Tonify qi/lung, Other: Move wei qi, Relieve itch) Lamiaceae/Labiatae
Cautions: Young children, Cardiac fibrillation, Epilepsy, Mucous membranes, Neurotoxic
Spearmint T/MC (Calm the shen, Release the exterior, Smooth liver qi, Spleen qi, Wei qi, Other: Relieve itch) Lamiaceae/Labiatae
Cautions: Neurotoxic, Pregnancy, Mucous membranes
Tangerine TC (Nourish blood, Move qi and blood, Spleen qi) Rutaceae
Cautions: May be photosensitive
Middle Warming...
Basil T/MW (Food stasis, Nourish yin/liver, Release the exterior, Spleen qi, Tonify qi//kidney, Tonify yang, Wei qi, Other: Promote lactation, Relieve uterine contraction) Lamiaceae/Labiatae
Cautions: Use in small doses, Pregnancy
Black Pepper MHot (Release exterior, Spleen qi, Tonify qi/kidney, Tonify yang, Wei qi) Piperacea
Cautions: Deficiency heat, Pregnancy
Caraway MW (Resolve damp phlegm, Spleen qi, Tonify qi, Other: Descend qi) Apiaceae/Umbelliferae
Cautions: Pregnancy, Children under 3, Cancer
Cardamom MW (Food stasis, Invigorate blood, Regulate qi, Spleen qi, Stop coughing, Tonify qi/Lung) Zingiberaceae
Cautions: Yin deficiency, Blood deficiency
Cinnamon Leaf MW (Invigorate blood, Release exterior, Spleen qi, Other: Promote sweating, Stimulate childbirth) Lauraceae
Cautions: Heat/empty heat
Coriander MW (Bi/expel wind damp cold, Nourish yin/liver, Spleen qi, Tonify qi/kidney, Wei qi) Apiaceae/Umbelliferae
Cautions: Pregnancy, Can be photosensitive
Cumin MsW (Invigorate blood, Smooth liver qi, Spleen qi, Tonify qi/heart) Apiaceae/Umbelliferae
Cautions: Photosensitive, Pregnancy
Fennel MW (Drain damp, Nourish yin, Spleen qi, Tonify qi/lung, Tonify yang) Apiaceae/Umbelliferae
Cautions: Estrogenic, Heat, Interior wind, Pregnancy, Cancer, Hypothyroidism
Ginger M/BHot (Invigorate blood, Parasites, Release exterior, Spleen qi, Tonify qi/lung/heart/kidney, Tonify yang, Warm interior to expel cold, Wei qi, Other: Harmonize blends) Zingiberaceae
Cautions: Heat/empty heat, Stomach fire

Hyssop MW(Bi/expel damp cold, Invigorate blood, Spleen qi, Tonify qi/lung/heart, Tonify yang) Lamiaceae/Labiatae
Cautions: Neurotoxic, Liver wind, Glaucoma, Cancer, Pregnancy, Children, Excessive use can cause asthma, seizures, hypertension
Juniper MW (Drain damp, Invigorate blood, Resolve phlegm, Spleen qi, Tonify yang/strongly, Other: Promote menstruation) Cupressaceae
Cautions: Kidney yin deficiency, Kidney toxicity, Pregnancy
Litsea MW (Bi/expel wind damp cold, Invigorate blood/lower, Regulate qi/lower, Release the exterior, Spleen qi, Tonify yang) Lauraceae
Cautions: Yin deficiency with heat
Nutmeg MW (Nourish blood, Move qi and blood, Spleen qi, Tonify yang/spleen/kidney, Warm interior to expel cold) Myristicaceae
Cautions: Diarrhea due to heat, Liver wind/ascending yang, Epilepsy, Liver toxicity, Pregnancy, High doses can produce delirium convulsions, Hallucinations, Dizziness, Fainting, Cancer
Oregano MW (Bi/expel wind damp cold, Move qi and blood, Open orifice, Parasites, Spleen qi, Wei qi, Other: Promotes menstruation) Lamiaceae/Labiatae
Cautions: Heat/empty heat, Pregnancy, Liver toxicity
Pennyroyal T/MW (Food stasis, Spleen qi, Stop coughing, Other: Promote bile, Regulate menses) Lamiaceae/Labiatae
Cautions: Pregnancy
Pine MW (Release the exterior, Resolve phlegm, Spleen qi, Stop cough, Tonify qi/lung/kidney, Tonify yang, Other: Descend qi to kidneys) Pinaceae
Cautions: Yin deficiency, Blood deficiency
Rosemary T/MW (Nourish blood, Regulate qi, Release the exterior, Spleen qi, Tonify qi/kidney/heart, Tonify yang, Warm the interior to expel cold) Lamiaceae/Labiatae
Cautions: Heat/empty heat, Pregnancy, Children, Rebellious qi, Hypertension
Savory MW (Nourish blood, Parasites, Resolve phlegm, Spleen qi, Tonify qi) Lamiaceae/Labiatae
Cautions: Heat/empty heat, Pregnancy
Tarragon MW (Food stasis, Moves qi and blood, Nourish Blood, Parasites, Spleen qi, Tonify Qi/heart, Other: Promote menstruation) Asteraceae
Cautions: Pregnancy, Cancer
Middle Neutral..
Geranium T/MN (Astringe/lower, Calm the shen, Cool the blood, Food stasis, Nourish yin, Parasites, Smooth liver qi, Spleen qi, Tonify qi/kidney, Other: Regulates menses) Gereniaceae
Cautions: Estrogenic, Pregnancy

Rosewood MN (Parasites, Regulate qi, Release the exterior, Smooth liver qi, Spleen qi, Tonify qi, Wei qi) Lauraceae

Middle Cooling...

Celery Seed MC (Bi/wind damp, Clear fire toxin, Drain damp, Food stasis, Nourish yin/liver, Regulate qi, Smooth liver qi, Spleen qi, Tonify qi/kidney) Apiaceae/Umbelliferae
Cautions: Estrogenic, Photosensitive, Pregnancy, Breastfeeding

Clary Sage MC (Clear heat/stomach, Cool the blood, Nourish yin, Smooth liver qi, Spleen qi, Subdue wind, Tonify qi/heart/lung, Other: Clear empty heat, Encourages labor, Regulates menses, Running piglet qi) Lamiaceae/Labiatae
Cautions: Estrogenic, Can be narcotic in larger doses, Cancer, Pregancy, Alcohol consumption

German Chamomile MC (Calm the shen, Clear heat/liver/stomach/heart, Drain Damp, Nourish yin/heart, Smoothes Liver Qi, Spleen qi, Subdue wind, Tonify qi/Lung) Asteraceae/Compositae

Ho Leaf MC (Release exterior, Resolve phlegm, Spleen qi, Other: Harmonize Blends) Lauraceae
Cautions: Yang deficiency

Neroli M/BC (Clear heat/Heart/fire toxin, Spleen qi, Tonify qi) Rutaceae
Niaouli MC (Bi/wind damp/lower, Invigorate blood, Parasites, Release the exterior, Spleen qi, Tonify qi/lung/kidney, Wei qi) Myrtaceae
Cautions: Pregnancy, Children

Peppermint T/MC (Clear heat, Open portals, Regulate qi, Release exterior, Smooth liver qi, Spleen qi, Tonify qi/lung, Other: Move wei qi, Relieve itch) Lamiaceae/Labiatae
Cautions: Young children, Cardiac fibrillation, Epilepsy, Mucous membranes, Neurotoxic

Spearmint T/MC (Calm the shen, Release the exterior, Smooth liver qi, Spleen qi, Wei qi, Other: Relieve itch) Lamiaceae/Labiatae
Cautions: Neurotoxic, Pregnancy, Mucous membranes

Yarrow MCold (Clear heat, Moves qi and blood, Smoothes liver qi, Spleen qi, Tonifies qi/heart/kidney, Other: Ascend spleen qi, Promote sweating) Asteracea/Compositae
Cautions: Neurotoxic, Children, Pregnancy, Ragweed allergy

Base Warming...

Angelica BW (Calm the shen, Invigorate blood, Nourish blood, Smooth liver qi, Spleen qi, Tonify qi/lung, Wei qi, Other: Ease cough, Expel phlegm, Open the diaphragm) Apiaceae/Umbelliferae
Cautions: Photosensitive, Pregnancy, Diabetes

Benzoin BW (Bi/expel damp cold, Drain damp/lower, Spleen qi, Stop coughing, Tonify yang/spleen, Other: Diffuse lung qi) Styracaceae
Cautions: Heat, Empty heat

Cinnamon BHot (Astringe/blood, Bi/expel wind damp, Drain damp, Invigorate blood, Nourish blood, Parasites, Spleen qi, Tonify qi, Tonify yang, Warm interior to expel cold, Wei qi, Other: Regulate menstruation) Lauraceae
Cautions: Heat/empty heat, Mucous membranes, Pregnancy, May sensitize skin, Kidney, Liver toxicity, May prevent coagulation

Dill BW (Drain damp, Food stasis, Invigorate blood, Spleen qi, Stop coughing, Other: Lactation, Promote bile secretion) Apiaceae/Umbelliferae
Cautions: Heat/empty heat, Yin deficiency, Liver wind/ascending yang, Pregnancy

Ginger M/BHot (Invigorate blood, Parasites, Release exterior, Spleen qi, Tonify qi/lung/heart/kidney, Tonify yang, Warm interior to expel cold, Wei qi, Other: Harmonize blends) Zingiberaceae
Cautions: Heat/empty heat, Stomach fire

Patchouli BsW (Clear summer heat, Release the exterior, Strongly tonify spleen qi, Other: Release suppressed emotion) Lamiaceae/Labiatae

Base Cooling...

Cedarwood BC (Clear heat/Lung, Dry damp/lower, Spleen qi, Tonify qi/lung, Tonify yang/kidney/spleen, Other: Relieve itch) Cupressaceae
Cautions: Pregnancy, Prepubescent children

Lovage BCold (Clear heat/stomach/kidney, Drain damp, Resolve phlegm, Spleen qi) Apiaceae/Umbelliferae
Cautions: Photosensitive, Toxic

Myrrh BC (Clear heat/Lung/Stomach, Dry damp, Move qi and blood, Spleen qi, Other: Promotes healing of wounds) Burseraceae
Cautions: Pregnancy, Uterine bleeding

Neroli M/BC (Clear heat/Heart/fire toxin, Spleen qi, Tonify qi) Rutaceae

Vetiver BC (Calm the Shen, Clear heat, Cool the blood, Invigorate blood, Nourish blood, Nourish yin, Smooth liver qi, Spleen qi, Tonify qi/heart) Gramineae

STOP COUGH

Top Warming...

Pennyroyal T/MW (Food stasis, Spleen qi, Stop coughing, Other: Promote bile, Regulate menses) Lamiaceae/Labiatae
Cautions: Pregnancy

Spruce T/MW (Bi/expel wind cold, Calm the shen, Stop coughing, Tonify qi, Tonify yang, Wei qi, Other: Helps kidneys graps lung qi) Pinaceae
Caution: May irritate the skin

Top Cooling...

Sweet Marjoram T/MC (Bi/expel damp hot, Clear heat/liver, Food stasis, Regulate qi, Release exterior, Smooth liver qi, Stop coughing) Lamiaceae/Labiatae
Cautions: Asthma, Pregnancy

Middle Warming...

Cardamom MW (Food stasis, Invigorate blood, Regulate qi, Spleen qi, Stop coughing, Tonify qi/Lung) Zingiberaceae
Cautions: Yin deficiency, Blood deficiency

Pennyroyal T/MW (Food stasis, Spleen qi, Stop coughing, Other: Promote bile, Regulate menses) Lamiaceae/Labiatae
Cautions: Pregnancy

Pine MW (Release the exterior, Resolve phlegm, Spleen qi, Stop cough, Tonify qi/lung/kidney, Tonify yang, Other: Descend qi to kidneys) Pinaceae
Cautions: Yin deficiency, Blood deficiency

Spruce T/MW (Bi/expel wind cold, Calm the shen, Stop coughing, Tonify qi, Tonify yang, Wei qi, Other: Helps kidneys graps lung qi) Pinaceae
Caution: May irritate the skin

Middle Cooling..

Anise MC (Clear heat, Food stagnation, Regulate qi, Smooth liver qi, Stop cough, Other: Promote lactation) Apiaceae/Umbelliferae
Cautions: Mild estrogenic, Yin deficiency, Cancer, Pregnancy

Cypress M/BsC (Astringe, Clear heat/lung, Move qi and blood, Stop coughing, Other: Ascend spleen qi, Assist kidney to grasp lung qi) Cupressaceae
Cautions: Hypertension, Cancer

Fir MC (Bi/expel damp hot, Clear heat, Dry damp/lower, Resolve phlegm/damp, Stop coughing, Tonify qi/lung, Other: Help kidneys grasp qi) Pinaceae

Sweet Marjoram T/MC (Bi/expel damp hot, Clear heat/liver, Food stasis, Regulate qi, Release exterior, Smooth liver qi, Stop coughing) Lamiaceae/Labiatae
Cautions: Asthma, Pregnancy

Base Warming...

Benzoin BW (Bi/expel damp cold, Drain damp/lower, Spleen qi, Stop coughing, Tonify yang/spleen, Other: Diffuse lung qi) Styracaceae
Cautions: Heat, Empty heat

Dill BW (Drain damp, Food stasis, Invigorate blood, Spleen qi, Stop coughing, Other: Lactation, Promote bile secretion) Apiaceae/Umbelliferae
Cautions: Heat/empty heat, Yin deficiency, Liver wind/ascending yang, Pregnancy

Base Cooling...

Cypress M/BsC (Astringe, Clear heat/lung, Move qi and blood, Stop coughing, Other: Ascend spleen qi, Assist kidney to grasp lung qi) Cupressaceae
Cautions: Hypertension, Cancer

Inula BsC (Clear heat/Lung, Drain/transform damp/upper, Stop coughing, Tonify qi/heart, Wei qi) Asteracea/Compositae
Cautions: Toxicity

SUBDUE WIND

Top Cooling...
Mandarin TC (Calm the Shen, Food stasis, Regulate qi, Spleen qi, Subdue wind) Rutaceae
Middle Warming..
Terebinth MW (Bi/expel wind damp cold, Release Exterior, Subdue wind) Pinaceae
Cautions: Yin deficiency/liver/kidney, Blood deficiency, Epilepsy
Middle Cooling..
Clary Sage MC (Clear heat/stomach, Cool the blood, Nourish yin, Smooth liver qi, Spleen qi, Subdue wind, Tonify qi/heart/lung, Other: Clear empty heat, Encourages labor, Regulates menses, Running piglet qi) Lamiaceae/Labiatae
Cautions: Estrogenic, Can be narcotic in larger doses, Cancer, Pregancy, Alcohol consumption
German Chamomile MC (Calm the shen, Clear heat/liver/stomach/heart, Drain Damp, Nourish yin/heart, Smoothes Liver Qi, Spleen qi, Subdue wind, Tonify qi/Lung) Asteraceae/Compositae
Roman Chamomille MC (Calm the Shen, Clear heat/liver, Nourish blood, Nourish yin/liver, Regulate qi, Smooth liver qi, Subdue wind) Asteraceae/Compositae
Cautions: Yang deficiency, Ragweed allergy
Base Warming...
Valerian BW (Nourish blood, Nourish yin, Parasites, Regulate Qi, Subdue wind, Tonifies Qi/heart, Tonify Yang/heart, Wei qi) Valerianaceae
Cautions: Qi deficiency, Yang deficiency, Pregnancy, Children
Base Cooling...
Spikenard BC (Calms the shen, Clear heat/Heart, Nourish yin/heart, Smooths liver qi, Subdue wind) Valerianaceae
Cautions: Exogenous conditions

TONIFY QI

Top Warming..

Ajowan Seed TW (Parasites, Spleen qi, Tonifies Qi/Lung, Tonify Yang, Wei qi)
Cautions: Pregnancy

Basil T/MW (Food stasis, Nourish yin/liver, Release the exterior, Spleen qi, Tonify qi//kidney, Tonify yang, Wei qi, Other: Promote lactation, Relieve uterine contraction) Lamiaceae/Labiatae
Cautions: Use in small doses, Pregnancy

Eucalyptus Radiata TW (Drain damp, Resolve Phlegm, Tonify qi, Wei qi) Myrtaceae

Rosemary T/MW (Nourish blood, Regulate qi, Release the exterior, Spleen qi, Tonify qi/kidney/heart, Tonify yang, Warm the interior to expel cold) Lamiaceae/Labiatae
Cautions: Heat/empty heat, Pregnancy, Children, Rebellious qi, Hypertension

Spruce T/MW (Bi/expel wind cold, Calm the shen, Stop coughing, Tonify qi, Tonify yang, Wei qi, Other: Helps kidneys graps lung qi) Pinaceae
Caution: May irritate the skin

Top Neutral..

Geranium T/MN (Astringe/lower, Calm the shen, Cool the blood, Food stasis, Nourish yin, Parasites, Smooth liver qi, Spleen qi, Tonify qi/kidney, Other: Regulates menses) Gereniaceae
Cautions: Estrogenic, Pregnancy

Top Cooling..

Blue Yarrow TC (Clear Heat, Moves qi and blood, Tonifies qi/heart)
Cautions: Pregnancy

Citronella TCold (Release the exterior, Tonify qi, Wei qi) Graminae
Cautions: Yang deficiency

Eucalyptus Smithii TC (Drain damp, Resolve Phlegm, Tonifies Qi, Wei qi) Myrtaceae
Cautions: Children 3 and under, Pregnancy

Lavender T/MC (Calm the Shen, Clear heat/lung/liver, Nourish yin, Parasites, Regulate qi, Release the exterior, Smooth liver qi, Tonify qi/heart, Tonify yang/heart, Other: Diffuse lung qi) Lamiaceae/Labiatae

Peppermint T/MC (Clear heat, Open portals, Regulate qi, Release exterior, Smooth liver qi, Spleen qi, Tonify qi/lung, Other: Move wei qi, Relieve itch) Lamiaceae/Labiatae
Cautions: Young children, Cardiac fibrillation, Epilepsy, Mucous membranes, Neurotoxic

Sage T/MC (Clear heat/stomach, Nourish yin, Release exterior, Resolve phlegm, Tonifies Qi/kidney, Other: Promote bile, Wei qi) Lamiaceae/Labiatae
Cautions: May be estrogenic, Seizures, Pregnancy, Tisserand recommends avoiding Sage in aromatherapy.
Middle Warming...

Basil T/MW (Food stasis, Nourish yin/liver, Release the exterior, Spleen qi, Tonify qi//kidney, Tonify yang, Wei qi, Other: Promote lactation, Relieve uterine contraction) Lamiaceae/Labiatae
Cautions: Use in small doses, Pregnancy

Black Pepper MHot (Release exterior, Spleen qi, Tonify qi/kidney, Tonify yang, Wei qi) Piperacea
Cautions: Deficiency heat, Pregnancy

Caraway MW (Resolve damp phlegm, Spleen qi, Tonify qi, Other: Descend qi) Apiaceae/Umbelliferae
Cautions: Pregnancy, Children under 3, Cancer

Cardamom MW (Food stasis, Invigorate blood, Regulate qi, Spleen qi, Stop coughing, Tonify qi/Lung) Zingiberaceae
Cautions: Yin deficiency, Blood deficiency

Coriander MW (Bi/expel wind damp cold, Nourish yin/liver, Spleen qi, Tonify qi/kidney, Wei qi) Apiaceae/Umbelliferae
Cautions: Pregnancy, Can be photosensitive

Cumin MsW (Invigorate blood, Smooth liver qi, Spleen qi, Tonify qi/heart) Apiaceae/Umbelliferae
Cautions: Photosensitive, Pregnancy

Fennel MW (Drain damp, Nourish yin, Spleen qi, Tonify qi/lung, Tonify yang) Apiaceae/Umbelliferae
Cautions: Estrogenic, Heat, Interior wind, Pregnancy, Cancer, Hypothyroidism

Ginger M/BHot (Invigorate blood, Parasites, Release exterior, Spleen qi, Tonify qi/lung/heart/kidney, Tonify yang, Warm interior to expel cold, Wei qi, Other: Harmonize blends) Zingiberaceae
Cautions: Heat/empty heat, Stomach fire

Hyssop MW(Bi/expel damp cold, Invigorate blood, Spleen qi, Tonify qi/lung/heart, Tonify yang) Lamiaceae/Labiatae
Cautions: Neurotoxic, Liver wind, Glaucoma, Cancer, Pregnancy, Children, Excessive use can cause asthma, seizures, hypertension

Pine MW (Release the exterior, Resolve phlegm, Spleen qi, Stop cough, Tonify qi/lung/kidney, Tonify yang, Other: Descend qi to kidneys) Pinaceae
Cautions: Yin deficiency, Blood deficiency

Rosemary T/MW (Nourish blood, Regulate qi, Release the exterior, Spleen qi, Tonify qi/kidney/heart, Tonify yang, Warm the interior to expel cold) Lamiaceae/Labiatae
Cautions: Heat/empty heat, Pregnancy, Children, Rebellious qi, Hypertension
Savory MW (Nourish blood, Parasites, Resolve phlegm, Spleen qi, Tonify qi) Lamiaceae/Labiatae
Cautions: Heat/empty heat, Pregnancy
Spruce T/MW (Bi/expel wind cold, Calm the shen, Stop coughing, Tonify qi, Tonify yang, Wei qi, Other: Helps kidneys graps lung qi) Pinaceae
Caution: May irritate the skin
Tarragon MW (Food stasis, Moves qi and blood, Nourish Blood, Parasites, Spleen qi, Tonify Qi/heart, Other: Promote menstruation) Asteraceae
Cautions: Pregnancy, Cancer
Middle Neutral...
Geranium T/MN (Astringe/lower, Calm the shen, Cool the blood, Food stasis, Nourish yin, Parasites, Smooth liver qi, Spleen qi, Tonify qi/kidney, Other: Regulates menses) Gereniaceae
Cautions: Estrogenic, Pregnancy
Rosewood MN (Parasites, Regulate qi, Release the exterior, Smooth liver qi, Spleen qi, Tonify qi, Wei qi) Lauraceae
Middle Cooling...
Cajeput MC (Bi/Expel damp hot, Drain damp/lower jiao, Move qi and blood, Parasites, Release exterior, Tonify qi/lung) Myrtaceae
Celery Seed MC (Bi/wind damp, Clear fire toxin, Drain damp, Food stasis, Nourish yin/liver, Regulate qi, Smooth liver qi, Spleen qi, Tonify qi/kidney) Apiaceae/Umbelliferae
Cautions: Estrogenic, Photosensitive, Pregnancy, Breastfeeding
Clary Sage MC (Clear heat/stomach, Cool the blood, Nourish yin, Smooth liver qi, Spleen qi, Subdue wind, Tonify qi/heart/lung, Other: Clear empty heat, Encourages labor, Regulates menses, Running piglet qi) Lamiaceae/Labiatae
Cautions: Estrogenic, Can be narcotic in larger doses, Cancer, Pregancy, Alcohol consumption
Fir MC (Bi/expel damp hot, Clear heat, Dry damp/lower, Resolve phlegm/damp, Stop coughing, Tonify qi/lung, Other: Help kidneys grasp qi) Pinaceae
Galbanum M/BC (Bi/expel damp hot, Calm the shen, Smooth liver qi, Tonify qi/lung,) Apiaceae/Umbelliferae
German Chamomile MC (Calm the shen, Clear heat/liver/stomach/heart, Drain Damp, Nourish yin/heart, Smoothes Liver Qi, Spleen qi, Subdue wind, Tonify qi/Lung) Asteraceae/Compositae

Inula BsC (Clear heat/Lung, Drain/transform damp/upper, Stop coughing, Tonify qi/heart, Wei qi) Asteracea/Compositae
Cautions: Toxicity

Lavender T/MC (Calm the Shen, Clear heat/lung/liver, Nourish yin, Parasites, Regulate qi, Release the exterior, Smooth liver qi, Tonify qi/heart, Tonify yang/heart, Other: Diffuse lung qi) Lamiaceae/Labiatae

Neroli M/BC (Clear heat/Heart/fire toxin, Spleen qi, Tonify qi) Rutaceae

Niaouli MC (Bi/wind damp/lower, Invigorate blood, Parasites, Release the exterior, Spleen qi, Tonify qi/lung/kidney, Wei qi) Myrtaceae
Cautions: Pregnancy, Children

Peppermint T/MC (Clear heat, Open portals, Regulate qi, Release exterior, Smooth liver qi, Spleen qi, Tonify qi/lung, Other: Move wei qi, Relieve itch) Lamiaceae/Labiatae
Cautions: Young children, Cardiac fibrillation, Epilepsy, Mucous membranes, Neurotoxic

Sage T/MC (Clear heat/stomach, Nourish yin, Release exterior, Resolve phlegm, Tonifies Qi/kidney, Other: Promote bile, Wei qi)
Lamiaceae/Labiatae
Cautions: May be estrogenic, Seizures, Pregnancy, Tisserand recommends avoiding Sage in aromatherapy.

Tea Tree MC (Clear heat, Dry damp, Invigorate blood, Parasites, Release exterior, Tonify qi, Wei qi) Myraceae

Thyme Linalool MC (Clear heat/lung/stomach, Parasites, Tonify qi) Lamiaceae/Labiatae
Cautions: Glaucoma

Yarrow MCold (Clear heat, Moves qi and blood, Smoothes liver qi, Spleen qi, Tonifies qi/heart/kidney, Other: Ascend spleen qi, Promote sweating) Asteracea/Compositae
Cautions: Neurotoxic, Children, Pregnancy, Ragweed allergy

Ylang Ylang M/BC (Calm the Shen, Clear heat/heart fire, Cool the blood, Nourish yin/heart/kidney, Tonifies qi/kidney, Wei qi) Annonaceae
Cautions: Yang deficiency, Cold

Base Warming...

Angelica BW (Calm the shen, Invigorate blood, Nourish blood, Smooth liver qi, Spleen qi, Tonify qi/lung, Wei qi, Other: Ease cough, Expel phlegm, Open the diaphragm) Apiaceae/Umbelliferae
Cautions: Photosensitive, Pregnancy, Diabetes

Balsam of Peru BW (Calm the Shen, Moves qi and blood, Parasites, Resolve phlegm, Tonifies Qi/Heart, Wei qi) Fabaceae
Cautions: May cause sensitization, Pregnancy, Breastfeeding

Cinnamon BHot (Astringe/blood, Bi/expel wind damp, Drain damp, Invigorate blood, Nourish blood, Parasites, Spleen qi, Tonify qi, Tonify yang, Warm interior to expel cold, Wei qi, Other: Regulate menstruation) Lauraceae
Cautions: Heat/empty heat, Mucous membranes, Pregnancy, May sensitize skin, Kidney, Liver toxicity, May prevent coagulation
Cistus BsW (Smooth liver qi, Tonify spleen, Other: Stop bleeding) Cistaceae
Cautions: Pregnancy
Ginger M/BHot (Invigorate blood, Parasites, Release exterior, Spleen qi, Tonify qi/lung/heart/kidney, Tonify yang, Warm interior to expel cold, Wei qi, Other: Harmonize blends) Zingiberaceae
Cautions: Heat/empty heat, Stomach fire
Valerian Root BW (Nourish blood, Nourish yin, Parasites, Regulate Qi, Subdue wind, Tonifies Qi/heart, Tonify Yang/heart, Wei qi) Valerianaceae
Cautions: Qi deficiency, Yang deficiency, Pregnancy, Children
Vanilla BsW (Calm the Shen, Tonify qi/kidney, Other: Release suppressed emotion) Orchidaceae
Base Cooling..
Cedarwood BC (Clear heat/Lung, Dry damp/lower, Spleen qi, Tonify qi/lung, Tonify yang/kidney/spleen, Other: Relieve itch) Cupressaceae
Cautions: Pregnancy, Prepubescent children
Frankincense BsCd (Calm the shen, Clear heat/Lung/Stomach, Dry damp, Nourish blood/liver, Resolve phlegm, Strongly move qi and blood, Tonify qi/lung, Other: Reduce swelling) Berceraceae
Cautions: Pregnancy
Galbanum M/BC (Bi/expel damp hot, Calm the shen, Smooth liver qi, Tonify qi/lung,) Apiaceae/Umbelliferae
Inula BsC (Clear heat/Lung, Drain/transform damp/upper, Stop coughing, Tonify qi/heart, Wei qi) Asteracea/Compositae
Cautions: Toxicity
Neroli M/BC (Clear heat/Heart/fire toxin, Spleen qi, Tonify qi) Rutaceae
Vetiver BC (Calm the Shen, Clear heat, Cool the blood, Invigorate blood, Nourish blood, Nourish yin, Smooth liver qi, Spleen qi, Tonify qi/heart) Gramineae
Violet BC (Calm the Shen, Clear heat/lung/fire toxin, Tonify qi/lung/heart, Other: Harmonize heart and kidney) Violaceae
Cautions: Yang deficiency, Cold
Ylang Ylang M/BC (Calm the Shen, Clear heat/heart fire, Cool the blood, Nourish yin/heart/kidney, Tonifies qi/kidney, Wei qi) Annonaceae
Cautions: Yang deficiency, Cold

TONIFY YANG

Top Warming...
Ajowan Seed TW (Parasites, Spleen qi, Tonifies Qi/Lung, Tonify Yang, Wei qi)
Cautions: Pregnancy
Basil T/MW (Food stasis, Nourish yin/liver, Release the exterior, Spleen qi, Tonify qi//kidney, Tonify yang, Wei qi, Other: Promote lactation, Relieve uterine contraction) Lamiaceae/Labiatae
Cautions: Use in small doses, Pregnancy
Clove THot (Parasites, Spleen qi, Tonify yang/kidney, Warm interior to expel cold) Myrtaceae
Cautions: Yin deficiency, Pregnancy, May prevent coagulation
Lemongrass TW (Nourish blood, Spleen qi, Tonify yang, Warm interior to expel cold, Wei qi) Graminae
Cautions: Heat/empty heat, Glaucoma, Children, Prostatic hyperplasia, Slight risk of sensitization
Rosemary T/MW (Nourish blood, Regulate qi, Release the exterior, Spleen qi, Tonify qi/kidney/heart, Tonify yang, Warm the interior to expel cold) Lamiaceae/Labiatae
Cautions: Heat/empty heat, Pregnancy, Children, Rebellious qi, Hypertension
Spruce T/MW (Bi/expel wind cold, Calm the shen, Stop coughing, Tonify qi, Tonify yang, Wei qi, Other: Helps kidneys graps lung qi) Pinaceae
Caution: May irritate the skin
Top Cooling...
Lavender T/MC (Calm the Shen, Clear heat/lung/liver, Nourish yin, Parasites, Regulate qi, Release the exterior, Smooth liver qi, Tonify qi/heart, Tonify yang/heart, Other: Diffuse lung qi) Lamiaceae/Labiatae
Middle Warming...
Basil T/MW (Food stasis, Nourish yin/liver, Release the exterior, Spleen qi, Tonify qi//kidney, Tonify yang, Wei qi, Other: Promote lactation, Relieve uterine contraction) Lamiaceae/Labiatae
Cautions: Use in small doses, Pregnancy
Black Pepper MHot (Release exterior, Spleen qi, Tonify qi/kidney, Tonify yang, Wei qi) Piperacea
Cautions: Deficiency heat, Pregnancy
Fennel MW (Drain damp, Nourish yin, Spleen qi, Tonify qi/lung, Tonify yang) Apiaceae/Umbelliferae
Cautions: Estrogenic, Heat, Interior wind, Pregnancy, Cancer, Hypothyroidism

Ginger M/BHot (Invigorate blood, Parasites, Release exterior, Spleen qi, Tonify qi/lung/heart/kidney, Tonify yang, Warm interior to expel cold, Wei qi, Other: Harmonize blends) Zingiberaceae
Cautions: Heat/empty heat, Stomach fire

Hyssop MW(Bi/expel damp cold, Invigorate blood, Spleen qi, Tonify qi/lung/heart, Tonify yang) Lamiaceae/Labiatae
Cautions: Neurotoxic, Liver wind, Glaucoma, Cancer, Pregnancy, Children, Excessive use can cause asthma, seizures, hypertension

Juniper MW (Drain damp, Invigorate blood, Resolve phlegm, Spleen qi, Tonify yang/strongly, Other: Promote menstruation) Cupressaceae
Cautions: Kidney yin deficiency, Kidney toxicity, Pregnancy

Litsea MW (Bi/expel wind damp cold, Invigorate blood/lower, Regulate qi/lower, Release the exterior, Spleen qi, Tonify yang) Lauraceae
Cautions: Yin deficiency with heat

Nutmeg MW (Nourish blood, Move qi and blood, Spleen qi, Tonify yang/spleen/kidney, Warm interior to expel cold) Myristicaceae
Cautions: Diarrhea due to heat, Liver wind/ascending yang, Epilepsy, Liver toxicity, Pregnancy, High doses can produce delirium convulsions, Hallucinations, Dizziness, Fainting, Cancer

Pine MW (Release the exterior, Resolve phlegm, Spleen qi, Stop cough, Tonify qi/lung/kidney, Tonify yang, Other: Descend qi to kidneys) Pinaceae
Cautions: Yin deficiency, Blood deficiency

Rosemary T/MW (Nourish blood, Regulate qi, Release the exterior, Spleen qi, Tonify qi/kidney/heart, Tonify yang, Warm the interior to expel cold) Lamiaceae/Labiatae
Cautions: Heat/empty heat, Pregnancy, Children, Rebellious qi, Hypertension

Spruce T/MW (Bi/expel wind cold, Calm the shen, Stop coughing, Tonify qi, Tonify yang, Wei qi, Other: Helps kidneys graps lung qi) Pinaceae
Caution: May irritate the skin

Middle Cooling..

Lavender T/MC (Calm the Shen, Clear heat/lung/liver, Nourish yin, Parasites, Regulate qi, Release the exterior, Smooth liver qi, Tonify qi/heart, Tonify yang/heart, Other: Diffuse lung qi) Lamiaceae/Labiatae

Base Warming..

Benzoin BW (Bi/expel damp cold, Drain damp/lower, Spleen qi, Stop coughing, Tonify yang/spleen, Other: Diffuse lung qi) Styracaceae
Cautions: Heat, Empty heat

Cinnamon BHot (Astringe/blood, Bi/expel wind damp, Drain damp, Invigorate blood, Nourish blood, Parasites, Spleen qi, Tonify qi, Tonify yang, Warm interior to expel cold, Wei qi, Other: Regulate menstruation) Lauraceae
Cautions: Heat/empty heat, Mucous membranes, Pregnancy, May sensitize skin, Kidney, Liver toxicity, May prevent coagulation
Ginger M/BHot (Invigorate blood, Parasites, Release exterior, Spleen qi, Tonify qi/lung/heart/kidney, Tonify yang, Warm interior to expel cold, Wei qi, Other: Harmonize blends) Zingiberaceae
Cautions: Heat/empty heat, Stomach fire
Valerian BW (Nourish blood, Nourish yin, Parasites, Regulate Qi, Subdue wind, Tonifies Qi/heart, Tonify Yang/heart, Wei qi) Valerianaceae
Cautions: Qi deficiency, Yang deficiency, Pregnancy, Children
Base Cooling...
Cedarwood BC (Clear heat/Lung, Dry damp/lower, Spleen qi, Tonify qi/lung, Tonify yang/kidney/spleen, Other: Relieve itch) Cupressaceae
Cautions: Pregnancy, Prepubescent children

WARM INTERIOR TO EXPEL COLD

Top Warming...
Clove THot (Parasites, Spleen qi, Tonify yang/kidney, Warm interior to expel cold) Myrtaceae
Cautions: Yin deficiency, Pregnancy, May prevent coagulation
Lemongrass TW (Nourish blood, Spleen qi, Tonify yang, Warm interior to expel cold, Wei qi) Graminae
Cautions: Heat/empty heat, Glaucoma, Children, Prostatic hyperplasia, Slight risk of sensitization
Rosemary T/MW (Nourish blood, Regulate qi, Release the exterior, Spleen qi, Tonify qi/kidney/heart, Tonify yang, Warm the interior to expel cold) Lamiaceae/Labiatae
Cautions: Heat/empty heat, Pregnancy, Children, Rebellious qi, Hypertension
Middle Warming...
Ginger M/BHot (Invigorate blood, Parasites, Release exterior, Spleen qi, Tonify qi/lung/heart/kidney, Tonify yang, Warm interior to expel cold, Wei qi, Other: Harmonize blends) Zingiberaceae
Cautions: Heat/empty heat, Stomach fire
Mugwort M/BW (Warm interior to expel cold, Other: Warm the uterus to promote menstruation) Asteraceae
Cautions: Heat/empty heat, Pregnancy, Neurotoxic
Nutmeg MW (Nourish blood, Move qi and blood, Spleen qi, Tonify yang/spleen/kidney, Warm interior to expel cold) Myristicaceae
Cautions: Diarrhea due to heat, Liver wind/ascending yang, Epilepsy, Liver toxicity, Pregnancy, High doses can produce delirium convulsions, Hallucinations, Dizziness, Fainting, Cancer
Onion MW (Invigorate blood, Parasites, Resolve phlegm, Warm interior to expel cold) Liliaceae
Cautions: Heat/empty heat
Rosemary T/MW (Nourish blood, Regulate qi, Release the exterior, Spleen qi, Tonify qi/kidney/heart, Tonify yang, Warm the interior to expel cold) Lamiaceae/Labiatae
Cautions: Heat/empty heat, Pregnancy, Children, Rebellious qi, Hypertension

Base Warming...

Cinnamon BHot (Astringe/blood, Bi/expel wind damp, Drain damp, Invigorate blood, Nourish blood, Parasites, Spleen qi, Tonify qi, Tonify yang, Warm interior to expel cold, Wei qi, Other: Regulate menstruation) Lauraceae

Cautions: Heat/empty heat, Mucous membranes, Pregnancy, May sensitize skin, Kidney, Liver toxicity, May prevent coagulation

Ginger M/BHot (Invigorate blood, Parasites, Release exterior, Spleen qi, Tonify qi/lung/heart/kidney, Tonify yang, Warm interior to expel cold, Wei qi, Other: Harmonize blends) Zingiberaceae

Cautions: Heat/empty heat, Stomach fire

Mugwort M/BW (Warm interior to expel cold, Other: Warm the uterus to promote menstruation) Asteraceae

Cautions: Heat/empty heat, Pregnancy, Neurotoxic

WEI QI

Top Warming..

Ajowan Seed TW (Parasites, Spleen qi, Tonifies Qi/Lung, Tonify Yang, Wei qi)
Cautions: Pregnancy

Basil T/MW (Food stasis, Nourish yin/liver, Release the exterior, Spleen qi, Tonify qi//kidney, Tonify yang, Wei qi, Other: Promote lactation, Relieve uterine contraction) Lamiaceae/Labiatae
Cautions: Use in small doses, Pregnancy

Eucalyptus Globulus T/MW (Drain damp, Move qi and blood, Parasites, Release the exterior, Wei qi) Myrtaceae
Cautions: Children and babies

Eucalyptus Radiata TW (Drain damp, Resolve Phlegm, Tonify qi, Wei qi) Myrtaceae

Lemongrass TW (Nourish blood, Spleen qi, Tonify yang, Warm interior to expel cold, Wei qi) Graminae
Cautions: Heat/empty heat, Glaucoma, Children, Prostatic hyperplasia, Slight risk of sensitization

Spruce T/MW (Bi/expel wind cold, Calm the shen, Stop coughing, Tonify qi, Tonify yang, Wei qi, Other: Helps kidneys graps lung qi) Pinaceae
Caution: May irritate the skin

Top Cooling...

Bergamot T/MsC (Clear heat/fire toxin, Drain damp, Food stagnation, Regulate qi, Release exterior, Smooth liver qi, Wei qi) Rutacae
Cautions: Photosensitive

Citronella TCold (Release the exterior, Tonify qi, Wei qi) Graminae
Cautions: Yang deficiency

Eucalyptus Citriodora TC (Drain damp, Move qi and blood, Wei qi,) Myrtaceae
Cautions: Children

Eucalyptus Smithii TC (Drain damp, Resolve Phlegm, Tonifies Qi, Wei qi) Myrtaceae
Cautions: Children 3 and under, Pregnancy

Lemon TCd (Bi/damp Invigorate blood, Clear heat/liver/GB/stomach, Spleen qi, Wei qi, Other: Break up stones) Rutaceae
Cautions: Photosensitive

Lime TC (Regulate qi/stomach/spleen, Wei qi, Other: Uplift mood) Rutaceae
Cautions: Photosensitive

Spearmint T/MC (Calm the shen, Release the exterior, Smooth liver qi, Spleen qi, Wei qi, Other: Relieve itch) Lamiaceae/Labiatae
Cautions: Neurotoxic, Pregnancy, Mucous membranes

Middle Warming..

Basil T/MW (Food stasis, Nourish yin/liver, Release the exterior, Spleen qi, Tonify qi//kidney, Tonify yang, Wei qi, Other: Promote lactation, Relieve uterine contraction) Lamiaceae/Labiatae
Cautions: Use in small doses, Pregnancy

Black Pepper MHot (Release exterior, Spleen qi, Tonify qi/kidney, Tonify yang, Wei qi) Piperacea
Cautions: Deficiency heat, Pregnancy

Coriander MW (Bi/expel wind damp cold, Nourish yin/liver, Spleen qi, Tonify qi/kidney, Wei qi) Apiaceae/Umbelliferae
Cautions: Pregnancy, Can be photosensitive

Eucalyptus Globulus T/MW (Drain damp, Move qi and blood, Parasites, Release the exterior, Wei qi) Myrtaceae
Cautions: Children and babies

Ginger M/BHot (Invigorate blood, Parasites, Release exterior, Spleen qi, Tonify qi/lung/heart/kidney, Tonify yang, Warm interior to expel cold, Wei qi, Other: Harmonize blends) Zingiberaceae
Cautions: Heat/empty heat, Stomach fire

Oregano MW (Bi/expel wind damp cold, Move qi and blood, Open orifice, Parasites, Spleen qi, Wei qi, Other: Promotes menstruation) Lamiaceae/Labiatae
Cautions: Heat/empty heat, Pregnancy, Liver toxicity

Spruce T/MW (Bi/expel wind cold, Calm the shen, Stop coughing, Tonify qi, Tonify yang, Wei qi, Other: Helps kidneys graps lung qi) Pinaceae
Caution: May irritate the skin

Middle Neutral..

Rosewood MN (Parasites, Regulate qi, Release the exterior, Smooth liver qi, Spleen qi, Tonify qi, Wei qi) Lauraceae

Middle Cooling..

Bergamot T/MsC (Clear heat/fire toxin, Drain damp, Food stagnation, Regulate qi, Release exterior, Smooth liver qi, Wei qi) Rutacae
Cautions: Photosensitive

Myrtle M/BCd (Astringe, Clear heat/Lung, Drain damp/lower, Smooth liver qi, Wei qi) Myrtaceae
Cautions: Yang deficiency, Cold

Niaouli MC (Bi/wind damp/lower, Invigorate blood, Parasites, Release the exterior, Spleen qi, Tonify qi/lung/kidney, Wei qi) Myrtaceae
Cautions: Pregnancy, Children

Spearmint T/MC (Calm the shen, Release the exterior, Smooth liver qi, Spleen qi, Wei qi, Other: Relieve itch) Lamiaceae/Labiatae
Cautions: Neurotoxic, Pregnancy, Mucous membranes

Tea Tree MC (Clear heat, Dry damp, Invigorate blood, Parasites, Release exterior, Tonify qi, Wei qi) Myraceae

Ylang Ylang M/BC (Calm the Shen, Clear heat/heart fire, Cool the blood, Nourish yin/heart/kidney, Tonifies qi/kidney, Wei qi) Annonaceae
Cautions: Yang deficiency, Cold
Base Warming...
Angelica BW (Calm the shen, Invigorate blood, Nourish blood, Smooth liver qi, Spleen qi, Tonify qi/lung, Wei qi, Other: Ease cough, Expel phlegm, Open the diaphragm) Apiaceae/Umbelliferae
Cautions: Photosensitive, Pregnancy, Diabetes
Cinnamon BHot (Astringe/blood, Bi/expel wind damp, Drain damp, Invigorate blood, Nourish blood, Parasites, Spleen qi, Tonify qi, Tonify yang, Warm interior to expel cold, Wei qi, Other: Regulate menstruation) Lauraceae
Cautions: Heat/empty heat, Mucous membranes, Pregnancy, May sensitize skin, Kidney, Liver toxicity, May prevent coagulation
Ginger M/BHot (Invigorate blood, Parasites, Release exterior, Spleen qi, Tonify qi/lung/heart/kidney, Tonify yang, Warm interior to expel cold, Wei qi, Other: Harmonize blends) Zingiberaceae
Cautions: Heat/empty heat, Stomach fire
Valerian BW (Nourish blood, Nourish yin, Parasites, Regulate Qi, Subdue wind, Tonifies Qi/heart, Tonify Yang/heart, Wei qi) Valerianaceae
Cautions: Qi deficiency, Yang deficiency, Pregnancy, Children
Base Cooling..
Helichrysum BC (Bi/expel damp hot, Clear heat/Lung/Liver/Fire Toxin, Cool the blood, Move qi and blood, Nourish blood, Smooth liver qi, Wei qi) Asteracea/Compositae
Cautions: Yang deficiency
Inula BsC (Clear heat/Lung, Drain/transform damp/upper, Stop coughing, Tonify qi/heart, Wei qi) Asteracea/Compositae
Cautions: Toxicity
Myrtle M/BCd (Astringe, Clear heat/Lung, Drain damp/lower, Smooth liver qi, Wei qi) Myrtaceae
Cautions: Yang deficiency, Cold
Ylang Ylang M/BC (Calm the Shen, Clear heat/heart fire, Cool the blood, Nourish yin/heart/kidney, Tonifies qi/kidney, Wei qi) Annonaceae
Cautions: Yang deficiency, Cold

Blends
Essential Oil Analogues of TCM Herbal Formulas

NOTE:

All dosages are the number of drops for 1/3 of an ounce of carrier oil.

Ba Zhen Tang

Blend 1
Tonify qi: Angelica
Nourish blood: Angelica, Frankincense
Regulate qi: Frankincense
Invigorate blood: Angelica, Frankincense
Spleen qi: Angelica
Dosages:
Angelica: 6
Frankincense: 4

Blend 2:
Tonify qi: Valerian
Nourish blood: Valerian
Regulate qi: Valarian, Myrrh
Invigorate blood: Myrrh
Spleen qi: Myrrh
Dosages:
Valerian: 5
Myrrh: 5

Suggested Points:
Tonify qi
Ren 17, Pc 6, St 36
Nourish blood
UB 17, Jiaji, Sp 3, 6, St 36, Kid 3
Regulate qi
LI 4, Liv 3
Invigorate blood
Sp 10, UB 17, Jiaji
Spleen qi
Sp 3, 4, 6

Technique:
Vibrating, Direction of meridian, Spiral

Suggested medium:
Olive

Frequency:
1xday

Ba Zheng San

Blend 1:
Clear heat: Helichrysum, Cedarwood
Drain damp: Cedarwood
Expel damp hot bi: Helichrysum
Spleen qi: Cedarwood
Dosages:
Helichrysum: 4
Cedarwood: 6

Blend 2:
Clear heat: Myrrh
Drain damp: Frankincense, Myrrh
Expel damp hot bi: Galbanum
Spleen qi: Myrrh
Dosages:
Frankincense: 4
Myrrh: 4
Galbanum: 2

Suggested Points:
Clear heat
LI 4, SJ 5, LI 11, Du 14
Drain damp
Sp 9, 3, 6, UB 20
Bi syndrome
LI 4, Liv 3, Sp 10, Ashi
Spleen qi
Sp 3, 4, 6

Technique:
Direction of Meridian, Vibrating, Spiral

Suggested medium:
Jojoba

Frequency:
1xday

Bai He Gu Jin Tang

Blend 1
Clear heat (lung) Lavendar
Nourish yin (lung, kidney) Lavendar
Resolve phlegm (lung) Ho Leaf
Dosage:
Lavender: 6 drops
Ho Leaf 3 drops

Blend 2
Clear heat (lung) Ravensare
Nourish yin (lung, kidney) Sage
Resolve phlegm (lung) Sage
Dosage:
Ravensare: 3 drops
Sage: 6 drops

Suggested Points:
Clear heat
LI 4, SJ 5, LI 11, Du 14
Nourish yin
Kid 3, UB 23, Ren 4, 6, Liv 3
Resolve phlegm
St 40, Sp 3, 6, 9

Technique:
Vibrating, Direction of meridian, Spiral, Vaporizer

Suggested medium:
Sesame

Frequency:
2xday

Bai Hu Tang

Blend 1:
Clear heat: Clary Sage
Nourish yin: Clary Sage
Dosage:
Clary Sage: 10

Blend 2:
Clear heat: Lavender
Nourish yin: Lavender
Dosage:
Lavender: 10

Suggested Points:
Clear heat
LI 4, SJ 5, LI 11, Du 14
Nourish yin
Kid 3, UB 23, Ren 4, 6, Liv 3

Technique:
Vibrating, Direction of meridian, Spiral

Suggested medium:
Sesame

Frequency:
2xday

Bai Tou Weng Tang

Blend 1:
Clear heat: Helichrysum
Cool the blood: Helichrysum
Drain damp: Cedarwood
Expel damp hot bi: Helichrysum
Dosage:
Helichrysum: 7 drops
Cedarwood: 3 drops

Blend 2:
Clear heat: Vetiver
Cool the blood: Vetiver
Drain damp: Lovage
Expel damp hot bi: Galbanum
Dosage:
Vetiver: 5
Lovage: 2
Galbanum: 3

Suggested Points:
Bi syndrome
LI 4, Liv 3, Sp 10, Ashi
Clear heat
LI 4, SJ 5, LI 11, Du 14
Cool the blood
Lu 9, Sp 10, LI 4, SJ 5, LI 11, Du 14
Drain damp
Sp 9, 3, 6, UB 20

Technique:
Vibrating, Direction of meridian, Spiral

Suggested medium:
Jojoba

Frequency:
1xday

Ban Xia Bai Zhu Tian Ma Tang

Blend 1:
Smooth liver qi: Helichrysum
Clear heat: Helichrysum, Jasmine
Invigorate blood: Helichrysum
Nourish yin: Jasmine
Subdue wind: Helichrysum (fire toxin), possibly add Roman Chamomille
Dosage:
Helichrysum: 6 drops
Jasmine: 4

Blend 2:
Smooth liver qi: Rose
Clear heat: Spikenard
Invigorate blood: Rose
Nourish yin: Rose,Spikenard
Subdue Wind: Spikenard
Dosage:
Spikenard: 6
Rose: 4

Suggested points:
Smooth liver qi
Liv 2(excess), Liv 3(deficiency), LI 4, Sp 6
Clear heat
LI 4, SJ 5, LI 11, Du 14
Invigorate blood
Sp 10, UB 17, Jiaji
Nourish yin
Kid 3, UB 23, Ren 4, 6, Liv 3
Subdue wind
Liv 3, Du 14, GB 20

Technique:
Vibrating, Direction of meridian, Spiral

Suggested medium:
Sesame

Frequency:
1xday

Ban Xia Hou Pu Tang

Blend 1:
Smooth liver qi: Clary Sage, Fir
Downbear/Regulate qi: Clary Sage (subdue wind), Fir
Resolve phlegm: Fir
Clear heat: Clary Sage, Fir
Dosages:
Fir: 6
Clary Sage: 4

Blend 2:
Smooth liver: Lavender
Downbear/Regulate qi: Lavender
Resolve phlegm: Sage
Clear heat: Lavender
Dosage:
Lavender: 8
Sage: 2

Suggested Points:
Smooth liver qi
Liv 2(excess), Liv 3(deficiency), LI 4, Sp 6
Regulate qi
LI 4, Liv 3
Resolve phlegm
St 40, Sp 3, 6, 9
Clear heat
LI 4, SJ 5, LI 11, Du 14

Technique:
Vibrating, Direction of meridian, Spiral

Suggested medium:
St. John's Wort

Frequency:
2xday

Ban Xia Xie Xin Tang

Blend 1:
Spleen qi: Celery Seed
Food stagnation: Celery Seed
Dosages:
Celery Seed: 10

Blend 2:
Spleen qi: Peppermint
Food stagnation: Sweet Marjoram (or possibly Melissa)
Dosages:
Peppermint: 5
Sweet Marjoram: 5

Suggested Points:
Spleen qi
Sp 3, 4, 6
Food stagnation
Ren 12, Pc 6, LI 4, Liv 3, St 25, 36, Sp 3

Technique:
Direction of meridian

Suggested medium:
Hazelnut

Frequency:
2xday

Bao He Wan

Blend 1:
Food stagnation: Anise
Spleen qi: Ho Leaf
Regulate qi: Anise
Clear heat: Anise
Resolve phlegm: Ho Leaf
Dosages:
Anise: 6
Ho Leaf: 4

Blend 2:
Food stagnation: Celery Seed
Tonify spleen: Celery Seed
Regulate qi: Celery Seed
Clear heat: Celery Seed
Resolve Phlegm: Sage
Dosages:
Celery Seed: 8
Sage: 2

Suggested Points:
Food stagnation
Ren 12, Pc 6, LI 4, Liv 3, St 25, 36, Sp 3
Spleen qi
Sp 3, 4, 6
Regulate qi
LI 4, Liv 3
Clear heat
LI 4, SJ 5, LI 11, Du 14
Resolve phlegm
St 40, Sp 3, 6, 9

Technique:
Direction of meridian, Spiral

Suggested medium:
Hazelnut

Frequency:
2xday

Bu Yang Huan Wu Tang

Blend 1:
Invigorate blood: Frankincense
Tonify qi: Frankincense
Dosage:
Frankincense: 10

Blend 2:
Move blood: Angelica
Tonify qi: Angelica
Dosage:
Angelica: 10

Suggested Points:
Invigorate blood
Sp 10, UB 17, Jiaji
Tonify qi
Ren 17, Pc 6, St 36

Technique:
Direction of meridian

Suggested medium:
Safflower

Frequency:
1xday

Bu Zhong Yi Qi Tang

Blend 1:
Spleen qi: Patchouli, Cinnamon
Tonify yang: Cinnamon
Dosage:
Cinnamon: 7
Patchouli: 3

Blend 2:
Spleen qi: Benzoin, Ginger
Tonify yang: Ginger Benzoin
Dosage:
Benzoin: 5
Ginger: 5

Suggested Points:
Spleen qi
Sp 3, 4, 6
Tonify yang
Du 4, St 36

Technique:
Direction of meridian

Suggested medium:
Hazelnut

Frequency:
1xday

Cang Er Zi San

Blend 1:
Clear heat: Palmarosa
Release exterior: Palmarosa
Resolve phlegm: Eucalyptus Smithii
Dosage:
Palmarosa: 6
Eucalyptus Smithii: 4

Blend 2:
Clear heat: Peppermint
Release exterior: Peppermint, Sage
Resolve phlegm: Sage
Dosage:
Peppermint: 5
Sage: 5

Suggested Points:
Clear heat
LI 4, SJ 5, LI 11, Du 14
Release the exterior
LI 4, SJ 5, LI 11, Du 14
Resolve phlegm
St 40, Sp 3, 6, 9, LI 20, Bitong, Yintang
NOTE: Halve dosage if used on the head.

Technique:
Spiral, Direction of meridian, Vaporizer

Suggested medium:
Sweet Almond

Frequency:
2xday

Chai Ge Jie Ji Tang

Blend 1:
Release exterior: Lavender, Niaouli
Bi syndrome: Niaouli
Clear heat: Lavender
Dosage:
Lavender: 5
Niaouli: 5

Blend 2:
Release exterior: Cajeput, Tea Tree
Bi sydrome: Cajeput
Clear heat: Tea Tree
Dosage:
Cajeput: 5
Tea Tree: 5

Suggested Points:
Release the exterior
LI 4, SJ 5, LI 11, Du 14
Bi syndrome
LI 4, Liv 3, Sp 10, Ashi
Clear heat
LI 4, SJ 5, LI 11, Du 14

Technique:
Spiral, Direction of meridian

Suggested medium:
Bitter Almond

Frequency:
2xday

Chai Hu Shu Gan San

Blend 1:
Smooth liver qi: Rose
Regulate qi: Frankincense
Invigorate blood: Frankincense, Rose
Dosage:
Rose: 5
Frankincense: 5

Blend 2:
Smooth liver qi: Helichrysum
Regulate qi: Helichrysum
Invigorate blood: Helichrysum
Dosage:
Helichrysum: 10

Suggested Points:
Smooth liver qi
Liv 2(excess), Liv 3(deficiency), LI 4, Sp 6
Regulate qi
LI 4, Liv 3
Invigorate blood
Sp 10, UB 17, Jiaji

Technique:
Vibrating, Direction of meridian

Suggested medium:
St. John's Wort

Frequency:
1xday

Chuan Xiong Cha Tiao San

Blend 1:
Release exterior: Eucalyptus Globlulus
Regulate qi: Eucalyptus Globlulus
Invigorate blood: Eucalyptus Globlulus
Dosage:
Eucalyptus Globulus: 10

Blend 2:
Release exterior: Rosemary
Regulate qi: Rosemary
Invigorate blood: Eucalyptus Citriodora
Dosage:
Rosemary: 5
Eucalyptus Citriodora: 5

Suggested points:
Release the exterior
LI 4, SJ 5, LI 11, Du 14
Regulate qi
LI 4, Liv 3
Invigorate blood
Sp 10, UB 17, Jiaji
Other
Yintang, Bitong, LI 20, GB 14
NOTE: Halve dosages if used on the head.

Technique:
Vibration, Spiral, Vaporizer

Suggested medium:
Bitter Almond

Frequency:
2xday

Da Bu Yin Wan

Blend 1:
Nourish yin: Rose
Clear empty heat: Rose, Roman Chamomille
Dosage:
Rose: 5
Roman Chamomille: 5

Blend 2:
Nourish yin: Ylang Ylang, German Chamomille
Clear empty heat: Ylang Ylang, German Chamomille
Dosages:
Ylang Ylang: 5
German Chamomille: 5

Suggested points:
Nourish yin
Kid 3, UB 23, Ren 4, 6, Liv 3
Clear heat
LI 4, SJ 5, LI 11, Du 14

Technique:
Vibrating, Spiral

Suggested medium:
Sesame

Frequency:
1xday

Da Chai Hu Tang

Blend 1:
Clear heat: Melissa
Release exterior: Melissa
Dosage:
Melissa: 10

Blend 2:
Clear heat: Lavender
Release exterior: Lavender
Dosage:
Lavender: 10

Suggested points:
Clear heat
LI 4, SJ 5, LI 11, Du 14
Release the exterior
LI 4, SJ 5, LI 11, Du 14

Technique:
Spiral

Suggested medium:
Sweet Almond

Frequency:
2xday

Da Cheng Qi Tang

Blend 1:
Cool lower jiao: Helichrysum
Regulate qi: Helichrysum
Dosage:
Helichrysum: 10

Blend 2:
Cool lower jiao: Sandalwood
Regulate qi: Frankincense
Dosages:
Sandalwood: 5
Frankincense: 5

Suggested points:
Clear heat
LI 4, SJ 5, LI 11, Du 14
Regulate qi
LI 4, Liv 3
Other:
St 25, 37

Technique:
Direction of meridian, Spiral

Suggested medium:
Jojoba

Frequency:
1xday

Da Jian Zhong Tang

Blend 1:
Spleen qi: Ginger, Oregano
Regulate qi: Oregano
Parasites: Ginger, Oregano
Dosages:
Ginger: 4
Oregano: 6

Blend 2:
Tonify spleen: Tarragon
Regulate qi: Tarragon
Parasiters: Tarragon
Dosage:
Tarragon: 10

Suggested Points:
Spleen qi
Sp 3, 4, 6
Regulate qi
LI 4, Liv 3
Parasites
St 25, Ren 4, LI 4

Techniques:
Vibrating, Direction of meridian

Suggested medium:
Walnut

Frequency:
2xday

Dang Gui Bu Xue Tang

Blend 1:
Nourish blood: Angelica
Tonify spleen: Angelica
Dosage:
Angelica: 10

Blend 2:
Nourish blood: Cinnamon
Tonify spleen: Patchouli
Dosage:
Cinnamon: 5
Patchouli: 5

Suggested Points:
Nourish blood
UB 17, Jiaji, Sp 3, 6, St 36, Kid 3
Spleen qi
Sp 3, 4, 6

Techniques:
Vibrating, Direction of meridian

Suggested medium:
Olive

Frequency:
1xday

Dang Gui Liu Huang Tang

Blend 1:
Nourish yin: Ylang Ylang
Tonify qi: Ylang Ylang
Nourish blood: Helichrysum
Clear heat: Ylang Ylang, Helichrysum
Dosage:
Ylang Ylang: 6
Helichrysum: 4

Blend 2:
Nourish yin: Vetiver
Tonify qi: Vetiver
Nourish blood: Vetiver
Clear heat: Vetiver
Dosage:
Vetiver: 10

Suggested Points:
Nourish yin
Kid 3, UB 23, Ren 4, 6, Liv 3
Tonify qi
Ren 17, Pc 6, St 36
Nourish blood
UB 17, Jiaji, Sp 3, 6, St 36, Kid 3
Clear heat
LI 4, SJ 5, LI 11, Du 14

Technique:
Vibrating, Direction of meridian, Spiral

Suggested medium:
Sesame

Frequency:
1xday

Dao Chi San

Blend 1:
Clear heart fire: German Chamomille
Nourish yin: German Chamomille
Dosage:
German Chamomille: 10

Blend 2:
Clear heart fire: Ylang Ylang
Nourish yin: Ylang Ylang
Dosage:
Ylang Ylang: 10

Suggested Points:
Clear heat
LI 4, SJ 5, LI 11, Du 14
Nourish yin
Kid 3, UB 23, Ren 4, 6, Liv 3

Technique:
Spiral, Vibrating

Suggested medium:
Sesame

Frequency:
2xday

Ding Chuan Tang

Blend 1:
Stop cough: Fir
Release exterior: Peppermint
Resolve phlegm: Fir
Dosage:
Fir: 6
Peppermint: 4

Blend 2:
Stop cough: Cypress
Release exterior: Sage
Resolve phlegm: Sage
Dosage:
Sage: 6
Cypress: 4

Suggested Points:
Stop cough
Ren 17, Lung 7
Release the exterior
LI 4, SJ 5, LI 11, Du 14
Resolve phlegm
St 40, Sp 3, 6, 9, Yintang, Bitong, LI 20
NOTE: Halve dosage for head.

Technique:
Spiral, Direction of meridian

Suggested medium:
Sweet Almond

Frequency:
2xday

Du Huo Ji Sheng Tang

Blend 1:
Bi syndrome: Cinnamon
Nourish yin: Rose
Tonify qi: Cinnamon
Nourish blood: Cinnamon
Dosage:
Cinnamon: 7
Rose: 3

Blend 2:
Bi syndrome: Styrax
Nourish yin: Vetiver
Tonify qi: Styrax
Nourish blood: Vetiver
Dosage:
Styrax: 6
Vetiver: 4

Suggested Points:
Bi syndrome
LI 4, Liv 3, Sp 10, Ashi
Nourish yin
Kid 3, UB 23, Ren 4, 6, Liv 3
Tonify qi
Ren 17, Pc 6, St 36
Nourish blood
UB 17, Jiaji, Sp 3, 6, St 36, Kid 3

Technique:
Vibrating, Direction of meridian

Suggested medium:
Walnut

Frequency:
1xday

Du Qi Wan

Blend 1:
Nourish yin: Ylang Ylang
Tonify qi: Frankincense
Assist kidney grasping qi: Cypress
Dosage:
Ylang Ylang: 4
Frankincense: 3
Cypress: 3

Blend 2:
Nourish yin: Rose
Tonify qi: Cedarwood
Assist kidney grasping qi: Benzoin
Dosage:
Rose: 4
Cedarwood: 3
Benzoin: 3

Suggested Points:
Nourish yin
Kid 3, UB 23, Ren 4, 6, Liv 3
Tonify qi
Ren 17, Pc 6, St 36
Kidneys grasping qi
Lung 7, Kid 6

Technique:
Vibrating, Direction of meridian

Suggested medium:
Hazelnut

Frequency:
1xday

Er Chen Tang

Blend 1 (warming)
Drain damp: Juniper
Resolve phlegm: Savory
Spleen qi: Savory
Food stagnation: Geranium
Dosage:
Juniper: 2
Geranium: 3
Savory: 5

Blend 2 (cooling)
Drain damp: German Chamomille
Phlegm: Caraway
Spleen: Caraway, German Chamomille
Food stagnation: Caraway (descend qi)
Dosage:
Caraway: 6
German Chamomille: 4

Suggested Points:
Drain damp
Sp 9, 3, 6, UB 20
Resolve phlegm
St 40, Sp 3, 6, 9
Spleen qi
Sp 3, 4, 6
Food stagnation
Ren 12, Pc 6, LI 4, Liv 3, St 25, 36, Sp 3

Technique:
Direction of meridian

Suggested medium:
Jojoba

Frequency:
2xday

Er Miao San

Blend 1:
Clear heat: Cedarwood
Drain damp: Cedarwood
Dosage:
Cedarwood: 10

Blend 2:
Clear heat: Lovage
Drain damp: Lovage
Dosage:
Lovage: 10

Suggested Points:
Clear heat
LI 4, SJ 5, LI 11, Du 14
Drain damp
Sp 9, 3, 6, UB 23

Technique:
Spiral, Direction of meridian

Suggested medium:
Jojoba

Frequency:
1xday

Er Xian Tang

Blend 1
Nourish yin: Rose
Tonify yang: Cinnamon
Regulate qi: Rose (smooth liver qi)
Dosage:
Rose: 6
Cinnamon: 4

Blend 2
Nourish yin: Ylang Ylang
Tonify yang: Ginger
Regulate qi: Cypress
Dosage:
Ylang Ylang: 4
Ginger: 4
Cypress: 2

Suggested Points:
Nourish yin
Kid 3, UB 23, Ren 4, 6, Liv 3
Tonify yang
Du 4, St 36
Regulate qi
LI 4, Liv 3

Technique:
Vibrate, Direction of meridian

Suggested medium:
Walnut

Frequency:
1xday

Er Zhi Wan

Blend 1
Nourish yin: Rose
Nourish blood: Helichrysum
Smooth liver qi: Rose, Helichrysum
Dosage:
Rose: 5
Helichrysum: 5

Blend 2
Nourish Yin: Vetiver
Nourish blood: Vetiver
Smooth liver qi: Vetiver
Dosage:
Vetiver: 10

Suggested Points:
Nourish yin
Kid 3, UB 23, Ren 4, 6, Liv 3
Nourish blood
UB 17, Jiaji, Sp 3, 6, St 36, Kid 3
Smooth liver qi
Liv 2(excess), Liv 3(deficiency), LI 4, Sp 6

Technique:
Vibrate, Direction of meridian

Suggested medium:
Sesame

Frequency
1xday

Fu Yuan Huo Xue Tang

Blend 1
Invigorate blood: Cinnamon Leaf
Regulate qi: Rosewood
Smooth liver qi: Rosewood
Dosage:
Rosewood: 6
Cinnamon Leaf: 4

Blend 2
Invigorate blood: Yarrow
Regulate qi: Yarrow
Smooth liver qi: Yarrow
Dosage:
Yarrow: 10

Suggested Points:
Invigorate blood
Sp 10, UB 17, Jiaji
Regulate qi
LI 4, Liv 3
Smooth liver qi
Liv 2(excess), Liv 3(deficiency), LI 4, Sp 6

Technique:
Direction of meridian

Suggested medium:
Safflower

Frequency:
2xday

Gan Mai Da Zao Tang

Blend 1
Nourish yin: Rose
Nourish qi: Balsam of Peru
Smooth liver qi: Rose
Dosage:
Rose: 6
Balsam of Peru: 4

Blend 2
Nourish yin: Valerian, Spikenard
Nourish qi: Valerian
Smooth liver qi: Spikenard
Dosage:
Valerian: 5
Spikenard: 5

Suggested points:
Nourish yin
Kid 3, UB 23, Ren 4, 6, Liv 3
Tonify qi
Ren 17, Pc 6, St 36
Smooth liver qi
Liv 2(excess), Liv 3(deficiency), LI 4, Sp 6

Technique:
Vibration, Direction of meridian

Suggested medium:
Hazelnut

Frequency:
1xday

Gan Mao Ling

Blend 1
Release exterior: Melissa
Clear heat: Melissa
Dosage:
Melissa: 10

Blend 2
Release exterior: Lavender
Clear heat: Lavender
Dosage:
Lavender: 10

Suggested Points:
Release the exterior
LI 4, SJ 5, LI 11, Du 14
Clear heat
LI 4, SJ 5, LI 11, Du 14

Technique:
Spiral, Vaporizer

Suggested medium:
Sweet Almond

Frequency:
2xday

Ge Gen Huang Lian Huang Qin Tang

Blend 1
Release exterior: Cajeput
Drain damp: Myrtle
Dosage:
Cajeput: 5
Myrtle: 5

Blend 2
Release exterior: Tea Tree
Drain damp: Tea Tree
Dosage:
Tea Tree: 10

Suggested Points:
Release the exterior
LI 4, SJ 5, LI 11, Du 14
Drain damp
Sp 9, 3, 6, UB 20

Technique:
Direction of meridian, Spiral

Suggested medium:
Sweet Almond

Frequency:
2xday

Ge Gen Tang

Blend 1
Release exterior (warming): Birch
Nourish yin: Fennel
Bi syndrome: Birch
Dosage:
Birch: 6
Fennel: 4

Blend 2
Release exterior (warming): Ginger
Nourish yin: Coriander
Bi syndrome: Coriander
Dosage:
Coriander: 6
Ginger: 4

Suggested Points:
Release the exterior
LI 4, SJ 5, LI 11, Du 14
Nourish yin
Kid 3, UB 23, Ren 4, 6, Liv 3
Bi syndrome
LI 4, Liv 3, Sp 10, Ashi

Technique:
Spiral, Vibrating, Direction of meridian

Suggested medium:
Sweet Almond

Frequency:
2xday

Ge Xia Zhu Yu Tang

Blend 1
Regulate qi: Angelica
Invigorate blood: Angelica, Rose
Nourish blood: Angelica
Smooth liver qi: Rose
Dosage:
Angelica: 6
Rose: 4

Blend 2
Regulate qi: Frankincense
Invigorate blood: Frankincense, Cinnamon
Nourish blood: Cinnamon
Smooth liver qi: Frankincense
Dosage:
Frankincense: 6
Cinnamon: 4

Suggested points:
Regulate qi
LI 4, Liv 3
Invigorate blood
Sp 10, UB 17, Jiaji
Nourish blood
UB 17, Jiaji, Sp 3, 6, St 36, Kid 3
Smooth liver qi
Liv 2(excess), Liv 3(deficiency), LI 4, Sp 6

Technique:
Vibrating, Direction of meridian

Suggested medium:
Safflower

Frequency:
1xday

Gui Pi Tang

Blend 1
Spleen qi: Angelica
Heart yin: Rose
Nourish blood: Angelica
Dosage:
Angelica: 6
Rose: 4

Blend 2
Spleen qi: Vetiver
Heart yin: Vetiver, Valerian
Nourish blood: Valerian
Dosage:
Vetiver: 5
Valerian: 5

Suggested Points:
Spleen qi
Sp 3, 4, 6
Nourish yin
Kid 3, UB 23, Ren 4, 6, Liv 3
Nourish blood
UB 17, Jiaji, Sp 3, 6, St 36, Kid 3

Suggested Medium:
Olive

Technique:
Vibrating, Direction of meridian

Frequency:
1xday

Gui Zhi Shao Yao Zhi Mu Tang

Blend 1:
Bi syndrome: Styrax
Drain damp: Benzoin
Regulate qi: Balsam of Peru
Dosage:
Styrax: 4
Benzoin: 3
Balsam of Peru: 3

Blend 2:
Bi syndrome: Cinnamon
Drain damp: Cinnamon
Regulate qi: Cypress
Dosage:
Cinnamon: 6
Cypress: 4

Suggested Points:
Bi syndrome
LI 4, Liv 3, Sp 10, Ashi
Drain damp
Sp 9, 3, 6, UB 20
Regulate qi
LI 4, Liv 3

Technique:
Direction of meridian

Suggested medium:
Walnut

Frequency:
1xday

Gui Zhi Tang

Blend 1
Release exterior: Wintergreen
Regulate qi: Ginger
Dosage:
Wintergreen: 5
Ginger: 5

Blend 2
Release exterior: Rosewood
Regulate qi: Rosewood
Warming: Cinnamon Leaf
Dosage:
Rosewood: 6
Cinnamon Leaf: 4

Suggested Points:
Release the exterior
LI 4, SJ 5, LI 11, Du 14
Regulate qi
LI 4, Liv 3
Other
Ren 17, Yintang, Bitong, LI 20
NOTE: Halve dosage if used on the head.

Technique:
Spiral, Direction of meridian

Suggested medium:
Sweet Almond

Frequency
2xday

Gui Zi Fu Ling Wan

Blend 1
Invigorate blood: Frankincense
Resolve phlegm: Frankincense
Regulate qi: Frankincense
Dosage:
Frankincense: 10

Blend 2:
Invigorate blood: Balsam of Peru
Resolve phlegm: Balsam of Peru
Regulate qi: Balsam of Peru
Dosage:
Balsam of Peru: 10

Suggested Points:
Invigorate blood
Sp 10, UB 17, Jiaji
Resolve phlegm
St 40, Sp 3, 6, 9
Regulate qi
LI 4, Liv 3

Technique:
Direction of meridian

Suggested medium:
Safflower

Frequency:
1xday

Huang Lian E Jiao Tang

Blend 1
Cool blood: Ylang Ylang
Nourish yin: Ylang Ylang
Clear fire: Ylang Ylang
Calm spirit: Ylang Ylang
Dosage:
Ylang Ylang: 10

Blend 2
Cool blood: Rose
Nourish yin: Rose, Spikenard
Clear fire: Spikenard
Calm spirit: Spikenard
Dosage:
Spikenard: 6
Rose: 4

Suggested Points:
Cool the blood
Lu 9, Sp 10, LI 4, SJ 5, LI 11, Du 14
Nourish yin
Kid 3, UB 23, Ren 4, 6, Liv 3
Clear heat
LI 4, SJ 5, LI 11, Du 14
Calm the shen
Pc 6, Du 20, Yintang
NOTE: Halve the dosage if used on the head

Technique:
Vibrating, Direction of meridian, Spiral

Suggested medium:
Sesame

Frequency:
1xday

Huang Lian Jie Du Tang

Blend 1
Clear heat: Helichrysum
Drain damp: Frankincense
Cool blood: Helichrysum
Dosage:
Helichrysum: 6
Frankincense: 4

Blend 2
Clear heat: Rose, Myrrh
Drain damp: Myrrh
Cool blood: Rose
Dosage:
Rose: 5
Myrrh: 5

Suggested Points:
Clear heat
LI 4, SJ 5, LI 11, Du 14
Drain damp
Sp 9, 3, 6, UB 20
Cool the blood
Lu 9, Sp 10, LI 4, SJ 5, LI 11, Du 14

Technique:
Spiral, Direction of meridian

Suggested medium:
Neem

Frequency:
1xday

Huo Xiang Zheng Qi Tang

Blend 1
Release the exterior: Cajeput, Naiouli
Drain damp: Cajeput
Regulate qi: Cajeput
Harmonize the middle: Niaouli
Dosage:
Cajeput: 6
Niaouli: 4

Blend 2
Release the exterior: Rosewood
Drain damp: German Chamomille
Regulate qi: Rosewood
Harmonize the middle: German Chamomille, Rosewood
Dosage:
Rosewood: 6
German Chamomille: 4

Suggested Points:
Release the exterior
LI 4, SJ 5, LI 11, Du 14
Drain damp
Sp 9, 3, 6, UB 20
Regulate qi
LI 4, Liv 3
Harmonize the middle:
Sp 3, 4, 6, Ren 12, St 36, Pc 6

Technique:
Spiral, Direction of meridian

Suggested medium:
Sweet Almond

Frequency:
2xday

Ji Chuan Jian

Blend 1
Tonify yang: Ginger
Nourish yin: Valerian
Regulate qi: Valerian
Dosage:
Valerian: 6
Ginger: 4

Blend 2
Tonify yang: Cinnamon
Nourish yin: Sandalwood
Regulate qi: Sandalwood
Dosage:
Sandalwood: 6
Cinnamon: 4

Suggested points:
Tonify yang
Du 4, St 36
Nourish yin
Kid 3, UB 23, Ren 4, 6, Liv 3
Regulate qi
LI 4, Liv 3

Technique:
Vibrate, Direction of meridian

Suggested medium:
Walnut

Frequency:
1xday

Jiao Ai Tang

Blend 1
Nourish blood: Angelica
Astringe blood: Angelica
Regulate qi: Frankincense
Invigorate blood: Frankincense
Dosage:
Angelica: 5
Frankincense: 5

Blend 2
Nourish blood: Cinnamon
Astringe blood: Cinnamon
Regulate qi: Myrrh
Invigorate blood: Cinnamon, Myrrh
Dosage:
Cinnamon: 6
Myrrh: 4

Suggested Points:
Nourish blood
UB 17, Jiaji, Sp 3, 6, St 36, Kid 3
Astringe
Sp 1, 3, Du 20
Regulate qi
LI 4, Liv 3
Invigorate blood
Sp 10, UB 17, Jiaji

Technique:
Vibrate, Direction of meridian

Suggested medium:
Olive

Frequency:
1xday

Jin Gui Shen Qi Wan

Blend 1
Tonify yang: Cinnamon
Nourish yin: Jasmine
Drain damp: Cinnamon
Dosage:
Cinnamon: 6
Jasmine: 4

Blend 2
Tonify yang: Valerian
Nourish yin: Valerian
Drain damp: Benzoin
Dosage:
Valerian: 6
Benzoin: 4

Suggested Points:
Tonify yang
Du 4, St 36
Nourish yin
Kid 3, UB 23, Ren 4, 6, Liv 3
Drain damp
Sp 9, 3, 6, UB 20

Technique:
Vibration, Direction of meridian

Suggested medium:
Walnut

Frequency:
1xday

Jin Suo Gu Jing Wan

Blend 1
Nourish yin: Ylang Ylang
Tonify yang: Ginger
Astringe: Cypress
Dosage:
Ylang Ylang: 4
Ginger: 4
Cypress: 2

Blend 2
Nourish yin: Rose
Tonify yang: Cinnamon
Astringe: Cinnamon
Dosage:
Cinnamon: 6
Rose: 3

Suggested Points:
Nourish yin
Kid 3, UB 23, Ren 4, 6, Liv 3
Tonify yang
Du 4, St 36
Astringe
Sp 1, 3, Du 20

Technique:
Vibration, Direction of meridian

Suggested medium:
Walnut

Frequency:
1xday

Ju Pi Zhu Ru Tang

Blend 1
Regulates qi: Geranium, Anise
Tonify qi: Geranium
Clear heat: Anise
Spleen qi: Geranium
Downbear qi: Geranium, Anise
Dosage:
Geranium: 6
Anise: 4

Blend 2
Regulates qi: Peppermint
Tonify qi: Celery Seed
Clear heat: Peppermint
Spleen qi: Peppermint
Downbear qi: Celery Seed
Dosage:
Peppermint: 6
Celery seed: 4

Suggested Points:
Regulate qi
LI 4, Liv 3
Tonify qi
Ren 17, Pc 6, St 36
Clear heat
LI 4, SJ 5, LI 11, Du 14
Spleen qi
Sp 3, 4, 6
Downbear qi:
Ren 12, 9, Pc 6, LI 4, Liv 3, St 25, 36, Sp 3

Technique:
Direction of meridian, Spiral

Suggested medium:
Hazelnut

Frequency:
2xday

Juan Bi Tang

Blend 1
Tonify qi: Ginger
Bi syndrome: Birch
Release the exterior: Birch
Dosage:
Birch: 6
Ginger: 4

Blend 2
Tonify qi: Spruce
Bi syndrome: Wintergreen, Spruce
Release the exterior: Wintergreen
Dosage:
Wintergreen: 5
Spruce: 5

Suggested Points:
Tonify qi
Ren 17, Pc 6, St 36
Bi syndrome
LI 4, Liv 3, Sp 10, Ashi
Release the exterior
LI 4, SJ 5, LI 11, Du 14

Technique:
Direction of meridian, Spiral

Suggested medium:
Emu

Frequency:
2xday

Li Zhong Wan

Blend 1
Spleen qi: Benzoin
Tonify yang: Benzoin
Dosage:
Benzoin: 10

Blend 2
Spleen qi: Ginger
Tonify yang: Ginger
Dosage:
Ginger: 10

Suggested points:
Spleen qi
Sp 3, 4, 6
Tonify yang
Du 4, St 36

Technique:
Direction of meridian

Suggested medium:
Walnut

Frequency:
1xday

Ling Gui Zhu Gan Tang

Blend 1
Resolve phlegm: Juniper
Spleen qi: Juniper
Drain damp: Juniper
Dosage:
Juniper: 10

Blend 2
Resolve phlegm: Caraway
Spleen qi: Caraway
Drain damp: Fennel
Dosage:
Caraway: 7
Fennel: 3

Suggested Points:
Resolve phlegm
St 40, Sp 3, 6, 9
Spleen qi
Sp 3, 4, 6
Drain damp
Sp 9, 3, 6, UB 20

Technique:
Direction of meridian

Suggested medium:
Sweet Almond

Frequency:
2xday

Ling Jiao Gou Teng Tang

Blend 1:
Smooth liver qi: Rose
Subdue wind: Valerian
Nourish yin: Rose
Dosage:
Rose: 6
Valerian: 4

Blend 2:
Smooth liver qi: Spikenard, Vetiver
Subdue wind: Spikenard
Nourish yin: Vetiver
Dosage:
Spikenard: 5
Vetiver: 5

Suggested points:
Smooth liver qi
Liv 2(excess), Liv 3(deficiency), LI 4, Sp6
Subdue wind
Liv 2, 3, Du 14, GB 20
Nourish yin
Kid 3, UB 23, Ren 4, 6, Liv 3

Technique:
Vibrate, Direction of meridian

Suggested medium:
St John's Wort

Frequency:
1xday

Liu Wei Di Huang Wan

Blend 1
Nourish yin: Rose
Clear deficiency heat: German Chamomille
Dosage:
Rose: 6
German Chamomille: 4

Blend 2
Nourish yin: Ylang Ylang
Clear deficiency heat: Roman Chamomille
Dosage:
Ylang Ylang: 6
Roman Chamomille: 4

Suggested Points:
Nourish yin
Kid 3, UB 23, Ren 4, 6, Liv 3
Clear heat
LI 4, SJ 5, LI 11, Du 14

Technique:
Vibrating, Spiral

Suggested medium:
Sesame

Frequency:
1xday

Long Dan Xie Gan Tang

Blend 1
Clear heat: Sandalwood
Drain damp: Sandalwood, Cedarwood
Dosage:
Sandalwood: 6
Cedarwood: 4

Blend 2
Clear heat: Helichrysum
Drain damp: Myrrh
Dosage:
Helichrysum: 5
Myrrh: 5

Suggested Points:
Clear heat
LI 4, SJ 5, LI 11, Du 14
Drain damp
Sp 9, 3, 6, UB 20

Technique:
Direction of meridian

Suggested medium:
Jojoba

Frequency:
1xday

Ma Huang Tang

Blend 1
Release exterior: Rosemary
Warm interior to expel cold: Rosemary
Tonify qi: Rosemary
Dosage:
Rosemary: 10

Blend 2
Release exterior: Eucalyptus Globulus
Warm interior to expel cold: Eucalyptus Globulus
Tonify qi: Eucalyptus Radiati
Dosage:
Eucalyptus Globlulus: 6
Eucalyptus Radiati: 4

Suggested Points:
Release the exterior
LI 4, SJ 5, LI 11, Du 14
Warm exterior to expel cold
Du 4, St 36, Ren 6
Tonify qi
Ren 17, Pc 6, St 36

Technique:
Direction of meridian, Vaporizor

Suggested medium:
Sweet Almond

Frequency:
Every 2-4hrs

Ma Xing Yi Gan Tang

Blend 1
Release exterior: Rosewood
Drain damp: German Chamomille
Clear heat: German Chamomille
Dosage:
German Chamomille: 6
Rosewood: 4

Blend 2
Release exterior: Tea Tree
Drain damp: Tea Tree
Clear heat: Tea Tree
Dosage:
Tea Tree: 10

Suggested points:
Release the exterior
LI 4, SJ 5, LI 11, Du 14
Drain damp
Sp 9, 3, 6, UB 20
Clear heat
LI 4, SJ 5, LI 11, Du 14

Technique:
Direction of meridian, Spiral, Vaporizer

Suggested medium:
Sweet Almond

Frequency:
2xday

Ma Xing Shi Gan Tang

Blend 1
Regulate qi: Rosewood
Clear heat: Fir
Stop coughing: Fir
Release the exterior: Rosewood
Dosage:
Rosewood: 5
Fir: 5

Blend 2
Regulate qi: Lavender
Clear heat: Cypress, Lavender
Stop coughing: Cypress
Release the exterior: Lavender
Dosage:
Lavender: 6
Cypress: 4

Suggested Points:
Regulate qi
LI 4, Liv 3
Clear heat
LI 4, SJ 5, LI 11, Du 14
Stop cough
Ren 17, Lung 7
Release the exterior
LI 4, SJ 5, LI 11, Du 14

Technique:
Direction of meridian, Spiral, Vaporizer

Suggested medium:
Sweet Almond

Frequency:
2xday

Ma Zi Ren Wan

Blend 1
Nourish yin: Rose
Clear heat: Rose
Regulate qi: Frankincense
Dosage:
Rose: 6
Frankincence: 4

Blend 2
Nourish yin: Ylang Ylang
Clear heat: Helichrysum
Regulate qi: Helichrysum
Dosage:
Helichrysum: 6
Ylang Ylang: 4

Suggested points:
Nourish yin
Kid 3, UB 23, Ren 4, 6, Liv 3
Clear heat
LI 4, SJ 5, LI 11, Du 14
Regulate qi
LI 4, Liv 3

Technique:
Vibrating, Spiral, Direction of meridian, Suppository

Suggested medium:
Sesame

Frequency:
1xday

Mai Men Dong Tang
(Possibly add something to clear heat.)

Blend 1
Nourish yin: Geranium
Stop cough: Fir
Dosage:
Geranium: 5
Fir: 5

Blend 2
Nourish yin: Clary Sage
Stop cough: Anise
Dosage:
Clary Sage: 5
Anise: 5

Suggested Points:
Nourish yin
Kid 3, UB 23, Ren 4, 6, Liv 3
Stop cough
Ren 17, Lung 7

Technique:
Vibrate, Direction of meridian, Vaporizer

Suggested medium:
Sweet Almond

Frequency:
2xday

Mu Li San

Blend 1
Nourish yin: Lavender
Tonify qi: Lavender
Dosage:
Lavender: 10

Blend 2:
Nourish yin: Geranium
Tonify qi: Geranium
Dosage:
Geranium: 10

Suggested Points:
Nourish yin
Kid 3, UB 23, Ren 4, 6, Liv 3
Tonify qi
Ren 17, Pc 6, St 36

Technique:
Vibrating, Direction of meridian

Suggested medium:
Hazelnut

Frequency:
2xday

Nuan Gan Jian

Blend 1
Tonify yang: Cinammon
Regulate qi: Balsam of Peru
Dosage:
Cinnamon: 5
Balsam of Peru: 5

Blend 2
Tonify yang: Ginger
Regulate qi: Valerian
Dosage:
Ginger: 5
Valerian: 5

Suggested Points:
Tonify yang
Du 4, St 36
Regulate qi
LI 4, Liv 3

Technique:
Direction of meridian, Fire on the mountain

Suggested medium:
Walnut

Frequency:
1xday

Ping Wei San

Blend 1
Spleen qi: Dill
Food stasis: Dill
Dosage:
Dill: 10

Blend 2
Spleen qi: Patchouli
Food stasis: Styrax
Dosage:
Patchouli: 5
Styrax: 5

Suggested points:
Spleen qi
Sp 3, 4, 6
Food stagnation
Ren 12, Pc 6, LI 4, Liv 3, St 25, 36, Sp 3

Technique:
Direction of meridian

Suggested medium:
Jojoba

Techniques:
1xday

Pu Ji Xiao Du Yin

Blend 1
Release exterior: Peppermint
Clear heat: Peppermint
Dosage:
Peppermint: 10

Blend 2
Release exterior: Melissa
Clear heat: Melissa
Dosage:
Melissa: 10

Suggested Points:
Release the exterior
LI 4, SJ 5, LI 11, Du 14
Clear heat
LI 4, SJ 5, LI 11, Du 14

Technique:
Spiral

Suggested medium:
Chamomille

Frequency:
2xday

Qi Ju Di Huang Wan

Blend 1:
Nourish yin (Liver): Rose
Dosage:
Rose: 10

Blend 2:
Nourish yin (Liver): Jasmine
Dosage:
Jasmine: 10

Suggested points:
Nourish yin
Kid 3, UB 23, Ren 4, 6, Liv 3
Other
Sp 3, 6, GB 37, St 36

Technique:
Vibrating, Direction of meridian

Suggested medium:
Sesame

Frequency:
1xday

Qiang Huo Sheng Shi Tang

Blend 1:
Bi syndrome: Cinnamon
Drain damp: Cinnamon
Dosage:
Cinnamon: 10

Blend 2:
Bi syndrome: Benzoin
Drain damp: Benzoin
Dosage:
Benzoin: 10

Suggested points:
Bi syndrome
LI 4, Liv 3, Sp 10, Ashi
Drain damp
Sp 9, 3, 6, UB 20

Technique:
Spiral,Direction of meridian

Suggested medium:
Jojoba

Frequency:
1xday

Qing Gu San

Blend 1
Nourish yin: Ylang Ylang
Clear heat: German Chamomille
Dosage:
Ylang Ylang: 6
German Chamomille: 4

Blend 2
Nourish yin: Rose
Clear heat: Roman Chamomille
Dosage:
Rose: 6
Roman Chamomille: 4

Suggested Points:
Nourish yin
Kid 3, UB 23, Ren 4, 6, Liv 3
Clear heat
LI 4, SJ 5, LI 11, Du 14

Technique:
Vibrating, Spiral

Suggested medium:
Sesame

Frequency:
1xday

Qing Hao Bie Jia Tang

Blend 1
Clear heat: Ylang Ylang
Nourish yin: Ylang Ylang
Dosage:
Ylang Ylang: 10

Blend 2
Clear heat: Spikenard
Nourish yin: Spikenard
Dosage:
Spikenard: 10

Suggested Points:
Nourish yin
Kid 3, UB 23, Ren 4, 6, Liv 3
Clear heat
LI 4, SJ 5, LI 11, Du 14

Technique:
Vibrating, Spiral

Suggested medium:
Sesame

Frequency:
1xday

Qing Qi Hua Tan Wan

Blend 1
Clear heat: Cypress
Resolve phlegm: Sage
Stop cough: Cypress
Dosage:
Cypress: 6
Sage: 4

Blend 2
Clear heat: Fir
Resolve phlegm: Fir
Stop cough: Fir
Dosage:
Fir: 10

Suggested points:
Clear heat
LI 4, SJ 5, LI 11, Du 14
Resolve phlegm
St 40, Sp 3, 6, 9
Stop cough
Ren 17, Lung 7

Technique:
Spiral, Direction of meridian

Suggested medium:
Sweet Almond

Frequency:
2xday

Qing Wei San

Blend 1
Clear heat: Sage
Cool blood: Melissa
Nourish yin: Sage
Dosage:
Sage: 6
Melissa: 4

Blend 2
Clear heat: German Chamomille
Cool blood: Ylang Ylang
Nourish yin: Ylang Ylang
Dosage:
Ylang Ylang: 6
German chamomille: 4

Suggested Points:
Clear heat
LI 4, SJ 5, LI 11, Du 14, Pc 6, Ren 12, St 36, 44
Cool the blood
Lu 9, Sp 10, LI 4, SJ 5, LI 11, Du 14
Nourish yin
Kid 3, UB 23, Ren 4, 6, Liv 3

Technique:
Vibrating, Spiral, Direction of meridian

Suggested medium:
Sesame

Frequency:
2xday

Qing Ying Tang

Blend 1
Nourish yin: Rose
Clear heat: Helichrysum
Invigorate blood: Rose, Helichrysum
Dosage:
Rose: 5
Helichrysum: 5

Blend 2
Nourish yin: Vetiver
Clear heat: Vetiver
Invigorate blood: Vetiver
Dosage:
Vetiver: 10

Suggested Points:
Nourish yin
Kid 3, UB 23, Ren 4, 6, Liv 3
Clear heat
LI 4, SJ 5, LI 11, Du 14
Invigorate blood
Sp 10, UB 17, Jiaji

Technique:
Vibrating, Spiral, Direction of meridian

Suggested medium:
Sesame

Frequency:
1xday

Qing Zao Jiu Fei Tang

Blend 1
Nourish yin: Lavender
Stop cough: Cypress
Dosage:
Lavender: 5
Cypress: 5

Blend 2
Nourish yin: Carrot
Stop cough: Anise
Dosage:
Carrot: 5
Anise: 5

Suggested Points:
Nourish yin
Kid 3, UB 23, Ren 4, 6, Liv 3
Stop cough
Ren 17, Lung 7

Technique:
Vibrating, Direction of meridian, Vaporizer

Suggested medium:
Sweet Almond

Frequency:
2xday

Ren Shen Bai Du San

Blend 1
Release exterior: Wintergreen, Pine
Tonify qi: Pine
Bi syndrome: Wintergreen
Dosage:
Wintergreen: 5
Pine: 5

Blend 2
Release exterior: Birch
Tonify qi: Rosemary
Bi syndrome: Birch
Dosage:
Birch: 6
Rosemary: 4

Suggested Points:
Release the exterior
LI 4, SJ 5, LI 11, Du 14
Tonify qi
Ren 17, Pc 6, St 36
Bi syndrome
LI 4, Liv 3, Sp 10, Ashi

Technique:
Spiral, Direction of meridian

Suggested medium:
Walnut

Frequency:
2xday

San Zi Yang Qin Tang

Blend 1
Phlegm: Pine
Stop cough : Pine
Regulate qi: Eucalyptus Globulus
Invigorate blood: Eucalyptus Globulus
Dosage:
Pine: 6
Eucalyptus Globulous: 4

Blend 2
Phlegm: Caraway
Stop cough : Cardamom, Caraway
Regulate qi: Cardamom
Invigorate blood: Cardamom
Dosage:
Cardamom: 6
Caraway: 4

Suggested Points:
Resolve phlegm
St 40, Sp 3, 6, 9
Stop cough
Ren 17, Lung 7
Regulate qi
LI 4, Liv 3
Invigorate blood
Sp 10, UB 17, Jiaji

Technique:
Direction of meridian

Suggested medium:
Sweet Almond

Frequency:
2xday

Sang Ju Yin

Blend 1
Release exterior: Peppermint
Clear heat: Peppermint, Fir
Stop cough: Fir
Dosage:
Peppermint: 5
Fir: 4

Blend 2
Release exterior: Lavender
Clear heat: Cypress, Lavender
Stop cough: Cypress
Dosage:
Lavender: 5
Cypress: 5

Suggested Points:
Release the exterior
LI 4, SJ 5, LI 11, Du 14
Clear heat
LI 4, SJ 5, LI 11, Du 14
Stop cough
Ren 17, Lung 7

Technique:
Spiral, Direction of meridian

Suggested medium:
Sweet Almond

Frequency:
2xday

Sang Piao Xiao San

Blend 1
Nourish yin: Ylang Ylang
Regulate qi: Frankincense
Tonify qi: Ylang Ylang
Nourish blood: Frankincense
Dosage:
Ylang Ylang: 5
Frankincense: 5

Blend 2
Nourish yin: Rose
Regulate qi: Valerian
Tonify qi: Valerian
Nourish blood: Valerian
Dosage:
Valerian: 6
Rose 4

Suggested Points:
Nourish yin
Kid 3, UB 23, Ren 4, 6, Liv 3
Regulate qi
LI 4, Liv 3
Tonify qi
Ren 17, Pc 6, St 36
Nourish blood
UB 17, Jiaji, Sp 3, 6, St 36, Kid 3

Technique:
Vibrating, Direction of meridian

Suggested medium:
Sesame

Frequency
1xday

Sang Xing Tang

Blend 1
Clear heat: Cypress, Lavender
Nourish yin: Lavender
Stop cough: Cypress
Dosage:
Lavender: 5
Cypress: 5

Blend 2
Clear heat: Anise
Nourish yin: Ylang Ylang
Stop cough: Anise
Dosage:
Anise: 6
Ylang Ylang: 5

Suggested Points:
Clear heat
LI 4, SJ 5, LI 11, Du 14
Nourish yin
Kid 3, UB 23, Ren 4, 6, Liv 3
Stop cough
Ren 17, Lung 7

Technique:
Spiral, Vibrating, Direction of meridian

Suggested medium:
Sweet Almond

Frequency:
2xday

Shao Fu Zhu Yu Tang

Blend 1
Invigorate blood: Cinnamon
Regulate qi: Valerian
Dosage:
Cinnamon: 6
Valerian: 4

Blend 2
Invigorate blood: Balsam of Peru
Regulate qi: Balsam of Peru
Dosage:
Balsam of Peru: 10

Suggested Points:
Invigorate blood
Sp 10, UB 17, Jiaji
Regulate qi
LI 4, Liv 3

Technique:
Direction of meridian

Suggested medium:
Safflower

Frequency:
1xday

Shao Yao Tang

Blend 1
Clear heat: Sandalwood
Invigorate blood: Sandalwood
Regulate qi: Sandalwood
Dosage:
Sandalwood: 10

Blend 2
Clear heat: Helichrysum
Invigorate blood: Helichrysum
Regulate qi: Helichrysum
Dosage:
Helichrysum: 10

Suggested Points:
Clear heat
LI 4, SJ 5, LI 11, Du 14
Invigorate blood
Sp 10, UB 17, Jiaji
Regulate qi
LI 4, Liv 3

Technique:
Spiral, Direction of meridian

Suggested medium:
Jojoba

Frequency:
1xday

Shen Ling Bai Zhu San

Blend 1
Spleen qi: Benzoin
Drain damp: Benzoin
Dosage:
Benzoin: 10

Blend 2
Spleen qi: Patchouli
Drain damp: Cinnamon
Dosage:
Patchouli: 5
Cinnamon: 5

Suggested Points:
Spleen qi
Sp 3, 4, 6
Drain damp
Sp 9, 3, 6, UB 20

Technique:
Direction of meridian

Suggested medium:
Jojoba

Frequency:
1xday

Shen Tong Zhu Yu Tang

Blend 1:
Regulate qi: Tarragon
Invigorate blood: Tarragon
Bi syndrome: Birch
Dosage:
Tarragon: 7
Birch: 3

Blend 2:
Regulate qi: Oregano
Invigorate blood: Oregano
Bi syndrome: Oregano
Dosage:
Oregano: 10

Suggested Points:
Regulate qi
LI 4, Liv 3
Invigorate blood
Sp 10, UB 17, Jiaji
Bi syndrome
LI 4, Liv 3, Sp 10, Ashi

Technique:
Direction of meridian

Suggested medium:
Safflower

Frequency:
2xday

Sheng Hua Tang

Blend 1
Invigorate blood: Balsam of Peru, Cinnamon, Rose
Regulate qi: Balsam of Peru
Nourish yin: Rose
Tonify yang: Cinnamon
Dosage:
Balsam of Peru: 3
Cinnamon: 4
Rose: 3

Blend 2
Invigorate blood: Ginger
Regulate qi: Sandalwood
Nourish yin: Sandalwood
Tonify yang: Ginger
Dosage:
Ginger: 5
Sandalwood: 5

Suggested Points:
Invigorate blood
Sp 10, UB 17, Jiaji
Regulate qi
LI 4, Liv 3
Nourish yin
Kid 3, UB 23, Ren 4, 6, Liv 3
Tonify yang
Du 4, St 36

Technique:
Vibrating, Direction of meridian

Suggested medium:
Safflower

Frequency:
1xday

Sheng Mai San

Blend 1
Nourish yin: Geranium
Tonify qi: Ginger
Dosage:
Geranium: 5
Ginger: 5

Blend 2
Nourish yin: Fennel
Tonify qi: Fennel
Dosage:
Fennel: 10

Suggested Points:
Nourish yin
Kid 3, UB 23, Ren 4, 6, Liv 3
Tonify qi
Ren 17, Pc 6, St 36

Technique:
Vibrating, Direction of meridian

Suggested medium:
Sweet Almond

Frequency:
2xday

Shi Quan Da Bu Tang

Blend 1
Nourish yin: Angelica
Tonify qi: Angelica
Tonify yang: Cinnamon
Spleen qi: Cinnamon
Dosage:
Angelica: 5
Cinnamon: 5

Blend 2
Nourish yin: Valerian
Tonify qi: Valerian
Tonify yang: Ginger
Spleen qi: Ginger
Dosage:
Valerian: 4
Ginger: 6

Suggested Points:
Nourish yin
Kid 3, UB 23, Ren 4, 6, Liv 3
Tonify qi
Ren 17, Pc 6, St 36
Tonify yang
Du 4, St 36
Spleen qi
Sp 3, 4, 6

Technique:
Vibrating, Direction of meridian

Suggested medium:
Hazelnut

Frequency:
1xday

Shi Xiao San

Blend 1
Invigorate blood: Frankincense
Regulate qi: Frankincense
Warming: Ginger
Dosage:
Frankincense: 6
Ginger: 4

Blend 2
Invigorate blood: Balsam of Peru
Regulate qi: Balsam of Peru
Dosage:
Balsam of Peru: 10

Suggested Points:
Invigorate blood
Sp 10, UB 17, Jiaji
Regulate qi
LI 4, Liv 3

Technique:
Direction of meridian

Suggested medium:
Safflower

Frequency
1xday

Si Jun Zi Tang

Blend 1
Tonify spleen: Angelica
Tonify qi: Angelica
drain damp: Cinnamon
Dosage:
Angelica: 6
Cinnamon: 4

Blend 2
Tonify spleen: Benzoin
Tonify qi: Ginger
drain damp: Benzoin
Dosage:
Benzoin: 6
Ginger: 4

Suggested Points:
Spleen qi
Sp 3, 4, 6
Tonify qi
Ren 17, Pc 6, St 36
Drain damp
Sp 9, 3, 6, UB 20

Technique:
Direction of meridian

Suggested medium:
Hazelnut

Frequency:
1xday

Si Ni San

Blend 1
Smooth liver qi: Rosewood
Tonify spleen: Rosewood
Release the exterior: Rosewood
Dosage:
Rosewood: 10

Blend 2
Smooth liver qi: Peppermint
Tonify spleen: Peppermint
Release the exterior: Peppermint
Dosage:
Peppermint: 10

Suggested Points:
Smooth liver qi
Liv 2(excess), Liv 3(deficiency), LI 4, Sp 6
Spleen qi
Sp 3, 4, 6
Release the exterior
LI 4, SJ 5, LI 11, Du 14

Technique:
Direction of meridian, Spiral

Suggested medium:
Hazelnut

Frequency:
2xday

Si Shen Wan

Blend 1
Tonify yang: Cinnamon
Spleen qi: Cinnamon
Dosage:
Cinnamon: 10

Blend 2
Tonify yang: Ginger
Spleen qi: Patchouli
Dosage:
Ginger: 5
Patchouli: 5

Suggested Points:
Tonify yang
Du 4, St 36
Spleen qi
Sp 3, 4, 6

Technique:
Direction of meridian

Suggested medium:
Walnut

Frequency:
1xday

Si Wu Tang

Blend 1
Nourish blood: Angelica
Invigorate blood: Angelica
Smooth liver qi: Angelica
Dosage:
Angelica: 10

Blend 2
Nourish blood: Cinnamon
Invigorate blood: Cinnamon
Smooth liver qi: Helichrysum
Dosage:
Cinnamon: 6
Helichrysum: 4

Suggested Points:
Nourish blood
UB 17, Jiaji, Sp 3, 6, St 36, Kid 3
Invigorate blood
Sp 10, UB 17, Jiaji
Smooth liver qi
Liv 2(excess), Liv 3(deficiency), LI 4, Sp 6

Technique:
Direction of meridian

Suggested medium:
Olive

Frequency:
1xday

Su Zi Jiang Qi Tang

Blend 1
Resolve phlegm: Styrax
Stop coughing: Benzoin
Tonify yang: Benzoin
Diffuse lung qi: Benzoin
Dosage:
Benzoin: 7
Styrax: 3

Blend 2
Resolve phlegm: Elemi
Stop coughing: Cypress
Tonify yang: Ginger
Kidneys grasp lung qi: Cypress
Dosage:
Cypress: 4
Ginger: 4
Elemi: 2

Suggested Points:
Resolve phlegm
St 40, Sp 3, 6, 9
Stop cough
Ren 17, Lung 7
Tonify yang
Du 4, St 36
Other
UB 13, 23, Ren 17

Technique:
Direction of meridian

Suggested medium:
Bitter Almond

Frequency:
1xday

Suan Zao Ren Tang

Blend 1
Nourish blood: Helichrysum
Clear heat: Helichrysum, Ylang Ylang
Calm the shen: Ylang Ylang
Nourish yin: Ylang Ylang
Dosage:
Ylang Ylang: 6
Helichrysum: 4

Blend 2
Nourish blood: Vetiver
Clear heat: Vetiver
Calm the shen: Vetiver
Nourish yin: Vetiver
Dosage:
Vetiver: 10

Suggested Points:
Invigorate blood
Sp 10, UB 17, Jiaji
Clear heat
LI 4, SJ 5, LI 11, Du 14
Calm the shen
Pc 6, Du 20, Yintang
Nourish yin
Kid 3, UB 23, Ren 4, 6, Liv 3

Technique:
Vibrating, Direction of meridian, Spiral

Suggested medium:
Olive

Frequency:
1xday

Tian Ma Gou Teng Yin

Blend 1
Subdue wind: Spikenard
Smooth liver qi: Spikenard, Rose
Calm the shen: Ylang Ylang
Clear heat: Ylang Ylang, Rose
Invigorate blood: Rose
Nourish yin: Ylang Ylang, Rose
Dosage:
Spikenard: 4
Rose: 3
Ylang Ylang: 3

Blend 2
Subdue wind: Valerian
Smooth liver qi: Vetiver
Calm the shen: Vetiver
Clear heat: Vetiver
Invigorate blood: Vetiver
Nourish yin: Valerian, Vetiver
Dosage:
Vetiver: 6
Valerian Root: 4

Suggested Points:
Subdue wind
Liv 3, Du 14, GB 20
Smooth liver qi
Liv 2(excess), Liv 3(deficiency), LI 4, Sp 6
Calm the shen
Pc 6, Du 20, Yintang
Clear heat
LI 4, SJ 5, LI 11, Du 14
Invigorate blood
Sp 10, UB 17, Jiaji
Nourish yin
Kid 3, UB 23, Ren 4, 6, Liv 3

Technique:
Vibrating, Spiral, Direction of meridian
Suggested medium:
Sesame
Frequency:
1xday

Tian Tai Wu Yao San

Blend 1
Regulate qi: Balsam of Peru
Tonify yang: Cinnamon
Smooth liver qi: Rose
Dosage:
Balsam of Peru: 3
Cinnamon: 4
Rose: 3

Blend 2
Regulate qi: Valerian
Tonify yang: Ginger
Smooth liver qi: Angelica
Dosage:
Valerian: 3
Ginger: 4
Angelica: 3

Suggested Points:
Regulate qi
LI 4, Liv 3
Tonify yang
Du 4, St 36
Smooth liver qi
Liv 2(excess), Liv 3(deficiency), LI 4, Sp 6

Technique:
Direction of meridian

Suggested medium:
Walnut

Frequency:
1xday

Tian Wang Bu Xin Dan

Blend 1
Nourish yin: Ylang Ylang
Nourish blood: Narcissus
Calm spirit: Ylang Ylang
Clear heat: Ylang Ylang
Harmonize heart and kidney: Narcissus
Dosage:
Ylang Ylang: 6
Narcissus: 4

Blend 2
Nourish yin: Rose, Vetiver
Nourish blood: Vetiver
Calm spirit: Rose, Vetiver
Clear heat: Rose, Vetiver
Harmonize heart and kidney: Rose
Dosage:
Vetiver: 6
Rose: 4

Suggested Points:
Nourish yin
Kid 3, UB 23, Ren 4, 6, Liv 3
Nourish blood
UB 17, Jiaji, Sp 3, 6, St 36, Kid 3
Calm the shen
Pc 6, Du 20, Yintang
Clear heat
LI 4, SJ 5, LI 11, Du 14

Technique:
Vibrating, Direction of meridian, Spiral

Suggested medium:
Sesame

Frequency:
1xday

Tiao Wei Cheng Qi Tang

Blend 1
Clear heat: Sandalwood
Regulate qi: Sandalwood
Dosage:
Sandalwood: 10

Blend 2
Clear heat: Frankincense
Regulate qi: Frankincense
Dosage:
Frankincense: 10

Blend 3
Clear heat: Helichrysum
Regulate qi: Helichrysum
Dosage:
Helichrysum: 10

Suggested Points:
Clear heat
LI 4, SJ 5, LI 11, Du 14
Regulate qi
LI 4, Liv 3

Technique:
Spiral, Direction of meridian

Suggested medium:
Castor

Frequency:
1xday

Tong Xie Yao Fang

Blend 1
Smooth liver qi: Frankincense
Tonify spleen: Myrrh
Drain damp: Myrrh
Dosage:
Frankincense: 3
Myrrh: 7

Blend 2
Smooth liver qi: Helichrysum
Tonify spleen: Lovage
Drain damp: Lovage
Dosage:
Helichrysum: 3
Lovage: 7

Suggested Points:
Smooth liver qi
Liv 2(excess), Liv 3(deficiency), LI 4, Sp 6
Spleen qi
Sp 3, 4, 6
Drain damp
Sp 9, 3, 6, UB 20

Technique:
Direction of meridian

Suggested medium:
Hazelnut

Frequency:
1xday

Wan Dai Tang

Blend 1
Tonify spleen: Patchouli
Drain damp: Cinnamon
Dosage:
Patchouli: 5
Cinnamon: 5

Blend 2
Tonify spleen: Benzoin
Drain damp: Benzoin
Dosage:
Benzoin: 10

Suggested Points:
Spleen qi
Sp 3, 4, 6
Drain damp
Sp 9, 3, 6, UB 20

Technique:
Direction of meridian

Suggested medium:
Jojoba

Frequency:
1xday

Wen Dan Tang

Blend 1
Regulate qi: Frankincense, Myrrh
Resolve phlegm: Frankincense
Spleen qi: Myrrh
Dosage:
Frankincense: 5
Myrrh: 5

Blend 2
Regulate qi: Helichrysum
Resolve phlegm: Lovage
Spleen qi: Lovage
Dosage:
Lovage: 6
Helichrysum: 4

Suggested Points:
Regulate qi
LI 4, Liv 3
Resolve phlegm
St 40, Sp 3, 6, 9
Spleen qi
Sp 3, 4, 6

Technique:
Direction of meridian

Suggested medium:
Jojoba

Frequency:
1xday

Wen Jing Tang

Blend 1
Tonify yang: Cinnamon
Nourish blood: Cinnamon
Invigorates blood: Cinnamon
Warm interior to expel cold: Cinnamon
Dosage:
Cinnamon: 10

Blend 2
Tonify yang: Ginger
Nourish blood: Angelica
Invigorates blood: Angelica
Warm interior to expel cold: Ginger
Dosage:
Ginger: 5
Angelica: 5

Suggested Points:
Tonify yang
Du 4, St 36
Nourish blood
UB 17, Jiaji, Sp 3, 6, St 36, Kid 3
Invigorate blood
Sp 10, UB 17, Jiaji
Warm interior to expel cold
Du 4, St 36, Ren 6

Technique:
Fire on the mountain, Direction of meridian

Suggested medium:
Walnut

Frequency:
1xday

Wu Ling San

Blend 1
Drain damp: Cinnamon
Spleen qi: Patchouli
Tonify yang: Cinnamon
Regulate qi: Balsam of Peru
Dosage:
Cinnamon: 4
Patchouli: 4
Balsam of Peru: 2

Blend 2
Drain damp: Benzoin
Spleen qi: Cypress
Tonify yang: Benzoin
Regulate qi: Cypress
Dosage:
Benzoin: 5
Cypress: 5

Suggested points:
Drain damp
Sp 9, 3, 6, UB 20
Spleen qi
Sp 3, 4, 6
Tonify yang
Du 4, St 36
Regulate qi
LI 4, Liv 3

Technique:
Direction of meridian

Suggested medium:
Jojoba

Frequency:
1xday

Wu Pi San

Blend 1
Drain damp: Benzoin
Tonify spleen: Benzoin
Regulate qi: Valerian
Dosage:
Benzoin: 7
Valerian: 3

Blend 2
Drain damp: Cinnamon
Tonify spleen: Cinnamon
Regulate qi: Balsam of Peru
Dosage:
Cinnamon: 6
Balsam of Peru: 4

Suggested Points:
Spleen qi
Sp 3, 4, 6
Drain damp
Sp 9, 3, 6, UB 20
Regulate qi
LI 4, Liv 3

Technique:
Direction of meridian

Suggested medium:
Jojoba

Frequency:
1xday

Wu Wei Xiao Du Yin

Blend 1
Clear heat: Helichrysum
Clear fire toxin: Helichrysum
Cool the blood: Helichrysum
Dosage:
Helichrysum: 10

Blend 2
Clear heat: Ylang Ylang
Clear fire toxin: Neroli
Cools the blood: Ylang Ylang
Dosage:
Ylang Ylang: 6
Neroli: 4

Suggested Points:
Clear heat
LI 4, SJ 5, LI 11, Du 14
Cool the blood
Lu 9, Sp 10, LI 4, SJ 5, LI 11, Du 14

Technique:
Spiral

Suggested medium:
Chamomille

Frequency:
1xday

Wu Zhu Yu Tang

Blend 1
Tonify yang: Basil
Sleen qi: Basil
Descend stomach qi: Basil
Dosage:
Basil: 10

Blend 2
Tonify yang: Ginger
Spleen qi: Ginger
Descend stomach qi: Cardamom
Dosage:
Ginger: 6
Cardamom: 4

Suggested Points:
Tonify yang
Du 4, St 36
Spleen qi
Sp 3, 4, 6
Food stagnation
Ren 12, Pc 6, LI 4, Liv 3, St 25, 36, Sp 3

Technique:
Direction of meridian

Suggested medium:
Hazelnut

Frequency:
2xday

Xiao Chai Hu Tang

Blend 1
Release the exterior: Rosewood
Tonify spleen: Clary Sage
Wei qi: Rosewood
Dosage:
Rosewood: 6
Clary Sage: 4

Blend 2
Release the exterior: Naiouli
Tonify spleen: Naiouli
Wei qi: Naouli
Dosage:
Naiouli: 10

Suggested Points:
Release the exterior
LI 4, SJ 5, LI 11, Du 14
Spleen qi
Sp 3, 4, 6

Technique:
Spiral, Direction of meridian

Suggested medium:
Jojoba

Frequency:
2xday

Xiao Cheng Qi Tang

Blend 1:
Clear heat: Helichrysum
Regulate Qi: Helichrysum
Dosage:
Helichrysum: 10

Blend 2:
Clear heat: Myrrh
Regulate Qi: Myrrh
Dosage:
Myrrh: 10

Suggested points:
Clear heat
LI 4, SJ 5, LI 11, Du 14
Regulate qi
LI 4, Liv 3

Technique:
Spiral, Direction of meridian

Medium:
Castor

Frequency:
1xday

Xiao Feng San

Blend 1
Release exterior: Tea Tree
Clear heat: Tea Tree
Drain damp: Tea Tree
Dosage:
Tea Tree: 10

Blend 2
Release exterior: Lavender
Clear heat: Lavender
Drain damp: German Chamomille
Dosage:
Lavender: 6
German Chamomille: 4

Suggested Points:
Release the exterior
LI 4, SJ 5, LI 11, Du 14
Clear heat
LI 4, SJ 5, LI 11, Du 14
Drain damp
Sp 9, 3, 6, UB 20

Technique:
Spiral, Direction of meridian

Suggested medium:
Jojoba

Frequency:
2xday

Xiao Jian Zhong Tang

Blend 1
Tonify spleen: Savory
Tonify qi: Savory
Nourish blood: Savory
Dosage:
Savory: 10

Blend 2
Tonify spleen: Ginger, Tarragon
Tonify qi: Ginger
Nourish blood: Tarragon
Dosage:
Ginger: 5
Tarragon: 5

Suggested Points:
Spleen qi
Sp 3, 4, 6
Tonify qi
Ren 17, Pc 6, St 36
Nourish blood
UB 17, Jiaji, Sp 3, 6, St 36, Kid 3

Technique:
Direction of meridian

Suggested medium:
Hazelnut

Frequency:
2xday

Xiao Qing Long Tang

Blend 1
Release exterior: Pine
Spleen qi: Pine
Stop coughing: Pine
Assist Kidney to grasp lung qi: Pine
Dosage:
Pine: 10

Blend 2
Release exterior: Ginger
Spleen qi: Ginger
Stop coughing: Cypress
Assist Kidney to grasp lung qi: Cypress
Dosage:
Ginger: 5
Cypress: 5

Suggested Points:
Release the exterior
LI 4, SJ 5, LI 11, Du 14
Spleen qi
Sp 3, 4, 6
Stop cough
Ren 17, Lung 7

Technique:
Spiral, Direction of meridian

Suggested medium:
Bitter Almond

Frequency:
2xday

Xiao Yao San

Blend 1
Smooth liver qi: Vetiver
Spleen qi: Vetiver
Nourish blood: Vetiver
Dosage:
Vetiver: 10

Blend 2
Smooth liver qi: Helichrysum
Spleen qi: Myrrh
Nourish blood: Helichrysum
Dosage:
Helichrysum: 6
Myrrh: 4

Suggested Points:
Smooth liver qi
Liv 2(excess), Liv 3(deficiency), LI 4, Sp 6
Spleen qi
Sp 3, 4, 6
Nourish blood
UB 17, Jiaji, Sp 3, 6, St 36, Kid 3

Technique:
Direction of meridian

Suggested medium:
St. John's Wort

Frequency:
1xday

Xie Bai San

Blend 1
Clear heat: Cypress
Stop coughing: Cypress
Dosage:
Cypress: 10

Blend 2
Clear heat: Fir
Stop coughing: Fir
Dosage:
Fir: 10

Suggested Points:
Clear heat
LI 4, SJ 5, LI 11, Du 14
Stop cough
Ren 17, Lung 7

Technique:
Direction of meridian

Suggested medium:
Sweet Almond

Frequency:
2xday

Xie Xin Tang

Blend 1
Clear heat: Celery Seed
Drain damp: Celery Seed
Regulate qi: Celery Seed
Dosage:
Celery Seed: 10

Blend 2
Clear heat: German Chamomille
Drain damp: German Chamomille
Regulate qi: Roman Chamomille
Dosage:
German Chamomille: 6
Roman Chamomille: 4

Suggested Points:
Clear heat
LI 4, SJ 5, LI 11, Du 14
Drain damp
Sp 9, 3, 6, UB 20
Regulate qi
LI 4, Liv 3

Technique:
Spiral, Direction of meridian

Suggested medium:
Jojoba

Frequency:
2xday

Xi Jiao Di Huang Tang

Blend 1:
Clear heat: Vetiver
Cool the blood: Vetiver
Invigorate blood: Vetiver
Dosage:
Vetiver: 10

Blend 2:
Clear heat: Helichrysum
Cool the blood: Helichrysum
Invigorate blood: Helichrysum
Dosage:
Helichrysum: 10

Suggested Points:
Clear heat
LI 4, SJ 5, LI 11, Du 14
Cool the blood
Lu 9, Sp 10, LI 4, SJ 5, LI 11, Du 14
Invigorate blood
Sp10, UB 17, Jiaji

Technique:
Spiral, Direction of meridian

Suggested medium:
Safflower

Frequency:
1xday

Xing Su San

Blend 1
Stop coughing: Spruce
Nourish yin: Rose
Resolve phlegm: Balsam of Peru
Dosage:
Spruce: 3
Rose: 3
Balsam of Peru: 3

Blend 2
Stop coughing: Benzoin
Nourish yin: Valerian
Resolve phlegm: Styrax
Dosage:
Benzoin: 3
Valerian: 3
Styrax: 3

Suggested Points:
Stop cough
Ren 17, Lung 7
Nourish yin
Kid 3, UB 23, Ren 4, 6, Liv 3
Resolve phlegm
St 40, Sp 3, 6, 9

Technique:
Vibrating, Direction of meridian

Suggested medium:
Sweet Almond

Frequency:
1xday

Xue Fu Zhu Yu Tang

Blend 1
Invigorate blood: Yarrow
Regulate qi: Yarrow
Smooth liver qi: Yarrow
Dosage:
Yarrow: 10

Blend 2
Invigorate blood: Cypress
Regulate qi: Peppermint
Smooth liver qi: Peppermint
Dosage:
Peppermint: 6
Cypress: 4

Suggested Points:
Invigorate blood
Sp 10, UB 17, Jiaji
Regulate qi
LI 4, Liv 3
Smooth liver qi
Liv 2(excess), Liv 3(deficiency), LI 4, Sp 6
Other
Pc6, Ht 4, 5, 6, 7

Technique:
Direction of meridian

Suggested medium:
Safflower

Frequency:
2xday

Yi Guan Jian

Blend 1
Nourish yin: Rose
Smooth liver qi: Rose
Dosage:
Rose: 10

Blend 2
Nourish yin: Vetiver
Smooth liver qi: Vetiver
Dosage:
Vetiver: 10

Suggested Points:
Nourish yin
Kid 3, UB 23, Ren 4, 6, Liv 3
Smooth liver qi
Liv 2(excess), Liv 3(deficiency), LI 4, Sp 6

Technique:
Vibrating, Direction of meridian

Suggested medium:
Sesame

Frequency:
1xday

Yin Chen Hao Tang

Blend 1
Clear toxic heat: Helichrysum
Drain damp: Myrrh
Dosage:
Helichrysum: 5
Myrrh: 5

Blend 2
Clear toxic heat: Rose
Drain damp: Sandalwood
Dosage:
Rose: 5
Sandalwood: 5

Suggested Points:
Clear heat
LI 4, SJ 5, LI 11, Du 14
Drain damp
Sp 9, 3, 6, UB 20

Technique:
Spiral, Direction of meridian

Suggested medium:
Jojoba

Frequency:
1xday

Yin Qiao San

Blend 1
Release exterior: Bergamot
Clear heat: Bergamot
Dosage:
Bergamot: 10

Blend 2
Release exterior: Peppermint
Clear heat: Peppermint
Dosage:
Peppermint: 10

Suggested Points:
Release the exterior
LI 4, SJ 5, LI 11, Du 14
Clear heat
LI 4, SJ 5, LI 11, Du 14

Technique:
Spiral, Vaporizer

Suggested medium:
Sweet Almond

Frequency:
2xday

You Gui Wan

Blend 1
Tonify yang: Cinnamon
Nourish yin: Ylang Ylang
Dosage:
Cinnamon: 5
Rose: 5

Blend 2
Tonify yang: Ginger
Nourish yin: Rose
Dosage:
Ginger: 5
Valerian: 5

Suggested Points:
Tonify yang
Du 4, St 36
Nourish yin
Kid 3, UB 23, Ren 4, 6, Liv 3

Technique:
Vibrating, Fire on the mountain, Direction of meridian

Suggested medium:
Walnut

Frequency:
1xday

You Gui Yin

Blend 1:
Nourish yin: Ylang Ylang
Tonify Yang: Cinnamon
Astringe: Cinnamon
Dosage:
Cinnamon: 5
Ylang Ylang: 5

Blend 2:
Nourish yin: Rose
Tonify Yang: Ginger
Astringe: Cypress
Dosage:
Rose: 5
Ginger: 3
Cypress: 2

Suggested Points:
Astringe
Sp 1, 3, Du 20
Nourish yin
Kid 3, UB 23, Ren 4, 6, Liv 3
Tonify yang
Du 4, St 36

Technique:
Vibrating, Direction of meridian

Suggested medium:
Sesame

Frequency:
1xday

Yu Nu Jian

Blend 1
Clear heat (stomach): Frankincense
Nourish yin: Rose
Dosage:
Frankincense: 5
Rose: 5

Blend 2
Clear heat (stomach): Myrrh
Nourish yin: Ylang Ylang
Dosage:
Myrrh: 5
Ylang Ylang: 5

Suggested Poins:
Clear heat
LI 4, SJ 5, LI 11, Du 14
Nourish yin
Kid 3, UB 23, Ren 4, 6, Liv 3

Technique:
Spiral, Vibrating

Suggested medium:
Sesame

Frequency:
1xday

Yu Ping Feng San

Blend 1
Wei qi: Eucalyptus Globulus
Release the exterior: Eucalyptus Globulus
Dosage:
Eucalyptus Globulus: 10 drops

Blend 2
Wei qi: Rosemary
Release the exterior: Rosemary
Dosage:
Rosemary: 10 drops

Blend 3:
Wei qi: Basil
Release the exterior: Basil
Dosage:
Basil: 10 drops

Suggested Points:
Wei qi
Lu 9, Ren 17, Sp 3
Release the exterior
LI 4, SJ 5, LI 11, Du 14

Technique:
Spiral

Suggested medium:
Sweet Almond

Frequency:
Every 2-4 hours

Yue Ju Wan

Blend 1
Regulate qi: Helichrysum
Move blood: Helichrysum, Vetiver
Smooth liver qi: Helichrysum, Vetiver
Spleen qi: Vetiver
Dosage:
Helichrysum: 5
Vetiver: 5

Blend 2
Regulate qi: Frankincense
Move blood: Frankincense
Smooth liver qi: Frankincense
Spleen qi: Myrrh
Dosage:
Frankincense: 7
Myrrh: 3

Suggested Points:
Regulate qi
LI 4, Liv 3
Invigorate blood
Sp 10, UB 17, Jiaji
Smooth liver qi
Liv 2(excess), Liv 3(deficiency), LI 4, Sp 6
Spleen qi
Sp 3, 4, 6

Technique:
Direction of meridian

Suggested medium:
Emu

Frequency:
1xday

Zhen Gan Xi Feng Tang

Blend 1
Smooth liver qi: Rose, Spikenard
Nourish yin: Rose
Subdue wind: Spikenard
Dosage:
Rose: 5
Spikenard: 5

Blend 2
Smooth liver qi: Helichrysum
Nourish yin: Jasmine
Subdue wind: Valerian
Dosage:
Valerian: 4
Helichrysum: 3
Jasmine: 3

Suggested Points:
Smooth liver qi
Liv 2(excess), Liv 3(deficiency), LI 4, Sp 6
Nourish yin
Kid 3, UB 23, Ren 4, 6, Liv 3
Subdue wind
Liv 3, Du 14, GB 20

Technique:
Vibrating, Direction of meridian

Suggested medium:
Chamomille

Frequency:
1xday

Zhen Wu Tang

Blend 1
Tonify spleen: Patchouli
Drain damp: Cinnamon
Tonify yang: Cinnamon
Dosage:
Cinnamon: 6
Patchouli: 4

Blend 2
Tonify spleen: Benzoin, Ginger
Drain damp: Benzoin
Tonify yang: Ginger
Dosage:
Ginger: 5
Benzoin: 5

Suggested Points:
Spleen qi
Sp 3, 4, 6
Drain damp
Sp 9, 3, 6, UB 20
Tonify yang
Du 4, St 36

Technique:
Direction of meridian,Fire on the mountain

Suggested medium:
Walnut

Frequency:
1xday

Zhi Bai Di Huang Tang

Blend 1
Nourish yin: Ylang Ylang
Clear heat: German Chamomille
Dosage:
Ylang Ylang: 6
German Chamomille: 4

Blend 2
Nourish yin: Rose
Clear heat: Roman Chamomille
Dosage:
Rose: 6
Roman Chamomille: 4

Suggested Points:
Nourish yin
Kid 3, UB 23, Ren 4, 6, Liv 3
Clear heat
LI 4, SJ 5, LI 11, Du 14

Technique:
Vibrating, Spiral

Suggested medium:
Sesame

Frequency:
1xday

Zhi Gan Cao Tang

Blend 1
Tonify qi: Ginger
Nourish blood: Ginger
Nourish yin: Rose
Dosage:
Rose: 6
Ginger: 4

Blend 2
Tonify qi: Valerian
Nourish blood: Valerian
Nourish yin: Valerian
Dosage:
Valerian Root: 10

Suggested Points:
Tonify qi
Ren 17, Pc 6, St 36
Nourish blood
UB 17, Jiaji, Sp 3, 6, St 36, Kid 3
Nourish yin
Kid 3, UB 23, Ren 4, 6, Liv 3
Other
Ht: 4, 5, 6, 7

Technique:
Vibrating, Direction of meridian

Suggested medium:
Hazelnut

Frequency:
1xday

Zhi Sou San

Blend 1
Stop cough: Pine
Release exterior: Pine
Resolve phlegm: Pine
Dosage:
Pine: 10

Blend 2
Stop cough: Spruce
Release exterior: Rosewood
Resolve phlegm: Juniper
Dosage:
Spruce: 4
Rosewood: 3
Juniper: 3

Suggested Points:
Stop cough
Ren 17, Lung 7
Release the exterior
LI 4, SJ 5, LI 11, Du 14
Resolve phlegm
St 40, Sp 3, 6, 9

Technique:
Direction of meridian, Spiral, Vaporizer

Suggested medium:
Sweet Almond

Frequency:
2xday

Zhu Ling Tang

Blend 1:
Drain damp: Sandalwood
Clear heat: Ylang Ylang
Nourish yin: Ylang Ylang
Dosage:
Sandalwood: 4
Ylang Ylang: 6

Blend 2:
Drain damp: Lovage
Clear heat: Lovage
Nourish yin: Rose
Dosage:
Lovage: 6
Rose: 4

Suggested points:
Drain damp
Sp 9, 3, 6, UB 20
Clear heat
LI 4, SJ 5, LI 11, Du 14
Nourish yin
Kid 3, UB 23, Ren 4, 6, Liv 3

Technique:
Vibrating, Spiral, Direction of meridian

Suggested medium:
Jojoba

Frequency:
1xday

Zhu Ye Shi Gao Tang

Blend 1:
Spleen qi: Yarrow
Tonify qi: Yarrow
Clear heat: Yarrow
Nourish yin: Ylang Ylang
Dosage:
Yarrow: 7
Ylang Ylang: 3

Blend 2:
Spleen qi: Peppermint
Tonify qi: Peppermint
Clear heat: Peppermint, Lavender
Nourish yin: Lavender
Dosage:
Peppermint: 6
Lavender: 4

Suggested points:
Spleen qi
Sp 3, 4, 6
Tonify qi
Ren 17, Pc 6, St 36
Clear heat
LI 4, SJ 5, LI 11, Du 14
Nourish yin
Kid 3, UB 23, Ren 4, 6, Liv 3

Technique:
Vibrating, Spiral,Direction of meridian

Suggested medium:
Hazelnut

Frequency:
2xday

Zou Gui Wan

Blend 1:
Nourish yin: Ylang Ylang
Nourish blood: Frankincense
Tonify qi (kidney): Ylang Ylang
Dosage:
Ylang Ylang: 6
Frankincense: 4

Blend 2:
Nourish yin: Vetiver
Nourish blood: Vetiver
Tonify qi (kidney): Vanilla
Dosage:
Vetiver: 6
Vanilla: 4

Suggested points:
Nourish yin
Kid 3, UB 23, Ren 4, 6, Liv 3
Nourish blood
UB 17, Jiaji, Sp 3, 6, St 36, Kid 3
Tonify qi
Ren 17, Pc 6, St 36

Technique:
Vibrating, Direction of meridian

Suggested medium:
Sesame

Frequency:
1xday

Zuo Jin Wan

Blend 1:
Smooth liver qi: Anise
Food stagnation: Anise
Clear heat: Anise
Dosage:
Anise: 10

Blend 2:
Smooth liver qi: Bergamot
Food stagnation: Bergamot
Clear heat: Bergamot
Dosage:
Bergamot: 10

Suggested points:
Smooth liver qi
Liv 2(excess), Liv 3(deficiency), LI 4, Sp 6
Food stagnation
Ren 12, Pc 6, LI 4, Liv 3, St 25, 36, Sp 3
Clear heat
LI 4, SJ 5, LI 11, Du 14

Technique:
Direction of meridian, Spiral

Suggested medium:
St. John's Wort

Frequency:
2xday

Bibliography

Bergstrom, W. Kent: **http://www.bubishi.com/**

Lan, Ma and Joel Wallach: **Passport to Aromatheraphy,** Wellness Publications, LLC (September 2005)

Lawless, Julie: **The Illustrated Encyclopedia of Essential Oils,** Element Books Ltd.; 2nd edition (December 25, 1995)

Price, Len and Price, Shirley: **Carrier Oils,** Riverhead (December 9, 2001)

Price, Shirley: **Aromatherapy for Babies and Children,** Thorsons (January 25, 1996)

Schnuaubelt, Kurt: **Advanced Aromatherapy,** Healing Arts Press; First Edition edition (May 1, 1998)

Schutes, J. and Weaver C: **Aromatherapy for Bodyworkers,** Prentice Hall; 1 edition (September 30, 2007)

Tisserand, Robert: **Essential Oil Safety,** Churchill Livingstone; 1 edition (January 15, 1995)

Willmont, Dennis: **http://www.willmountain.com/**

Yuen, Jeffrey: **Materia Medica of Essential Oils from a TCM Standpoint,** Self-Published

Yuen, Jeffrey audio and video presentations from www.conferencerecording.com
  -Audio Recording: **Application of Essential Oils on Acupuncture Points,** 3 cd set
  -Audio Recording: **Application of Essential Oils on Acupuncture Points,** 1 cd
  -**Essential oils and Meditative States and TCM Face Reading,** 6 DVD set

Appendix: Chemical Constituents of Essential Oils

You can break down the oils into their chemical constituents, but you cannot synthesize them. You can combine chemicals together, but you cannot derive essential oils in that way. We believe this is because essential oils contain the living, vital essence of the plant. To be sure, this vital jing essence is comprised of chemical substances, but it is also imbued with refined, powerful life energy. It is this healing energy that cannot be artificially contrived or engineered in a lab and hence, makes their action so unique.

Here, we give a brief overview of the chemical substances. For much more indepth analysis, see:
Chemistry of Essential Oils by **David Stewart, The Healing Intelligence of Essential Oils** by **Kurt Schnaubelt, The Chemistry of Aromatherapeutic Oils** by **E. Joy Bowles,** and **The Chemistry of Essential Oils** by **David Williams**.

Alcohols: These tend to be very antiseptic and volatile.

Aldehydes: These are usually found in lemon scented oils. They tend to have a function of opening the orifice and calming the shen.

Esters: Esters are very common in plant essences. They are anti-fungal, anti-microbial and tend to have a fruity fragrance.

Ketones: Some ketones may be toxic, although there are some which do not have a toxic effect, such as those found in Jasmine. They can be useful in the treatment of wounds, however they should be used with care in the case of pregnant women.

Oxides: Oxides are great expectorants. Camphorous oils will tend to contain Oxides.

Phenols: Phenols are strong anti-microbials. However, they should not be used for long periods of time, as they can irritate skin and mucous membranes. They are great stimulants, but can also build up toxicity if used over time.

Terpenes: These constituents have a wide range of different effects, from analgesics to stimulants and decongestants. However they also tend to evaporate quickly.

www.ingramcontent.com/pod-product-compliance
Lightning Source LLC
Chambersburg PA
CBHW031830170526
45157CB00001B/249

* 9 7 8 1 4 8 1 9 7 3 4 8 9 *